How to Be

Healthy

Body, Mind, and Spirit

Dr. Lauren Deville

www.drlaurendeville.com

Lauren Deville

Lauren Deville

Information contained in this book is intended to inform and educate, and is not intended to be a substitution for individualized advice from a qualified medical professional. Readers are highly encouraged to seek a naturopathic physician in his or her neighborhood.

Published By: Wanderlust Publishing, Tucson, AZ

Table of Contents

Introduction

This book is designed to be a simple guide to better health, based on the following premise:

If you give your body what it needs to heal itself and remove the obstacles to cure, healing will follow.

This is the basic principle on which I practice medicine. How simple or how complicated the interpretation of this principle becomes in a given case depends on a couple of main variables:

1) How many obstacles to cure are present,

2) How many building blocks are missing,

3) How long the patient has been in the present condition, and/or

4) How willing the patient is to make the necessary changes.

Nature Cure is not easy (the more of the four variables you have against you, the harder it becomes), but it *is* usually easy to understand. Our bodies are designed to heal themselves. The physician's job is not to "make someone well," but rather to facilitate the process of healing. Most common ailments and diseases of the Western World will respond to this approach—even those that are supposedly governed by genetics. Most so-called "genetic" conditions are multifactorial (in other words, more than one gene contributes to the inheritance pattern, and we don't even necessarily know what they all are), and our environments determine which genes get turned on and turned off anyway. The exceptions to this are rare genetic mutation illnesses such as Multiple Sclerosis and Cystic Fibrosis, or conditions in which the damage is already so complete that the body no longer has the ability to self-correct, such as in Type 1 Diabetes or Addison's Disease. In these cases, long-term symptom management really is the most appropriate course of action. But those cases are much more rare than the first set.

Part One of this book is a broad-strokes overview, in which I tell four patient cases to illustrate the simplicity and harmony of these principles. While patient stories are different from one another, there are only so many obstacles to cure, and there are only so many building blocks that a given patient might be lacking. The job of the physician is to listen well, and identify the ones that are most appropriate in a case.

Part Two is about the building blocks to achieve

or maintain good health, and you can probably guess most of them: healthy food, good digestion, water, fresh air, sunlight, sleep, exercise, rest and relaxation, solid relationships, and a sense of peace and life purpose. Eliminate any one of them and you're asking for trouble. It's only a matter of time before the lack of it will take its toll on your health.

Part Three addresses common obstacles to cure. These range from poor food choices, to solvents, pesticides, mold exposure, and heavy metals; too many pharmaceuticals for too long (the side effects do add up), and stress in the form of poor time management, poor relationships, a poor self-image, or a job you hate. Over time these obstacles may create enough damage that you'll need some outside help to fix them before the body will be able to heal on its own.

The most common system dysfunctions I have seen are an unhealthy gut (*so* many issues go back to the gut), immune system dysfunction (either allergies or autoimmunity), adrenal fatigue, and hormonal imbalance. Many patients who have been ill for a long time present with more than one of these system dysfunctions, and sometimes all four.

It will almost certainly take time, patience, and lifestyle changes—but given the right environment, the right tools, and the appropriate mindset, you can reach your own personal optimal level of health.

1

PART 1:

REMOVING the Obstacles

and Supplying the Building

Blocks

Case 1:

"I'm a mess, aren't I? Have you ever seen a case as bad as mine before?"

Janice, a 38-year old new patient, said this to me at our first visit. I just laughed, and said, "Do you know how many people ask me that question?"

We'd just finished talking about the therapeutic order we would need to follow in order to restore her health. Janice presented with IBS (Irritable Bowel Syndrome), joint pain, weight gain, fatigue, and insomnia, and because so many systems are interrelated, I told her we'd need to address several of these at the same time. I sent her home with a diet diary to determine whether she had food sensitivities (which would require testing), candida overgrowth, or whether she simply made poor food choices. I gave her a salivary cortisol test kit to determine exactly how poorly her adrenals were functioning—I knew they were a problem, I just didn't know how much of a problem yet. I also gave her some Adrenal Support for some immediate relief of her fatigue, while we waited for the results to come back. I sent her for basic lab work, and did a complete thyroid workup as well, just because that's such a common cause of fatigue as well. Then again, so is insomnia—I gave her some glycine to help her get into the deeper stages of sleep so she wouldn't wake multiple times every night, and recommended a wind-down routine to help her turn her thoughts off before bedtime.

She'd written on her new patient paperwork that she worked 50-60 hours per week, as the manager of a restaurant. She described herself as a driven perfectionist, and rolled her eyes when she told the story of how many doctors in the past had told her, "You've got to manage your stress! You've got to start exercising!" Her response to this was a sarcastic, "Okay, great. You want to pay my bills? You want to call me in the morning and tell me to get my butt in the gym?"

But as Janice and I continued to talk, I recognized a few underlying beliefs which were limiting her ability to heal. She wasn't very nice to herself. Instead of recognizing her own value as a person, she didn't stop to acknowledge her own successes. Her internal voice was consistently harsh and condemning, driving her to work harder and accomplish more. As a result, she told me self-care was always last on her priority list—because she didn't value herself very highly. I knew it was unlikely that this would change without direct intervention at the level of the limiting belief: *that* was the root that led to the fruit of poor self-care and eventually, poor health.

So I gave her a handout to help her identify the most important tasks in her work day, and instructed her to use it to re-structure her work schedule such that she had five more hours per week to dedicate to self-care. I told her to get a coach online to keep her accountable for small changes, so she could have an external form of discipline until she was able to internalize it for herself. But I also asked her to start each day with a simple verbal affirmation: "I love and accept myself exactly as I am." I told her that takes between 21-30 days to build a new habit; if she was faithful to tell herself this every day, and be vigilant to stop the thoughts to the contrary when she recognized them, then in roughly that length of time she would actually change her belief. From that new seed, better fruit would follow.

This is the process of finding the root cause of an illness. It's usually a lot simpler than we think.

Janice returned three weeks later, already with more energy and sleeping much better. She had indeed cut back her work schedule by five hours per week (her boss was all for it, having lovingly accused her of perfectionism for years). She'd even started going to the gym once per week, with the help of her coach checking in on her via text daily.

One look at her diet diary confirmed what her lab work also told me: she had candida overgrowth. I put her on a 6 week candida protocol including a diet, natural antifungals, and probiotics, and I also sent her home with a symptom diary to track whether the joint pain and IBS improved entirely on this protocol, or only partially (indicating that we would need to investigate food allergies after all).

When she saw the food restrictions on the diet, Janice grimaced, asking how on earth she'd find time to prepare all her meals in order to stick to it.

"Well, I recommend a cookbook to help give you ideas," I told her. "But it's important to plan ahead, you're right. So pencil it in on your calendar every Sunday or whenever your weekend is, to plan your meals and shop for the week. Make large batches of whatever you'll need that evening, so you can eat on it all week long, and supplement the rest with salads or a few variations on a simple dish of meat, veggies, and whole grains."

When she still looked unconvinced, I added, "Bonus: I can virtually promise you'll lose weight on this!"

That sold her.

Janice's salivary cortisol test showed that her adrenal function was quite low, but with an inverted rhythm, meaning she had a spike of cortisol in the evenings. Her wind-down routine had helped, and she was sleeping through the night now, but she told me she still would lie awake for a good 30 minutes to an hour before finally drifting off. I treated this with phosphatidylserine, an extract of sunflowers, to blunt the cortisol spike such that she would fall asleep faster.

The rest of Janice's lab work looked good, except for subclinical hypothyroidism. Her TSH was high normal, at least according to the labs (3.3), while her free T4 and free T3 were both low normal. I told her it was possible that as we treated her adrenals, her thyroid might "wake up" and function better—or we might have to consider doing some natural thyroid (NatureThroid is my preference for most patients). She opted for the watch and wait approach.

Six weeks later, Janice returned having lost 11 pounds. Her gas, bloating, alternating constipation and diarrhea were gone. Her joint pain had vanished. Her insomnia was resolved, and her energy had jumped from 3/10 to 8/10, with no midday energy dip anymore. She'd increased her exercise to three days per week, and found that since her energy had increased, it wasn't nearly as big a chore to get herself to work out anymore.

"My coach isn't trying to get me to go to the gym anymore," she told me. "Now I just have him check in to make sure I'm not cheating on my diet!"

After that I transitioned her to a healthy general diet plan—and since she'd been so strict of the previous 6 weeks, the transition was actually a piece of cake (no pun intended).

Putting it Together:

Janice first needed to *subtract her obstacles to cure*. In her case, they were an unhealthy gut (Chapter 14), exhausted adrenals (Chapter 16), and limiting beliefs (Chapter 18)—on the surface her belief was "I don't have time," but just beneath that was "I'm not worth it."

Once we'd addressed those, she needed to *add the building blocks for health that she lacked*: sleep (Chapter 5), exercise (Chapter 6), rest and relaxation (Chapter 7), appropriate macronutrients (Chapter 1) and the ability to absorb her micronutrients (Chapter

2)—which followed naturally as soon as her gut healed.

Case 2

Patricia came to me with a bizarre rash, food sensitivities to nearly everything, and crushing fatigue, despite being on more than a full thyroid replacement dose, and more than a full adrenal replacement dose of hydrocortisone.

"When did this all start?" I asked her.

She and her husband thought for awhile, but finally she said, "About two years ago. That was the first time the rash showed up."

"Did anything change in your life two years ago?" I asked.

"We moved into a new house."

Ah. "Brand new?" I asked, flipping to the part of the new patient paperwork where she listed her chemical sensitivities. Sure enough, she'd indicated "very severe" on almost everything.

"No, but we gutted it," her husband said. "We ripped out the carpet, painted the walls, and did a bunch of renovation."

"My guess is, it was a solvent toxicity that did it," I told them. "Many paints contain VOCs, or Volatile Organic Compounds, and there are lots of things like flame retardants and other solvents in all the rest of the stuff you'd use for renovation."

The name of the game was to detox her and heal up her gut so that she could start absorbing her nutrients again, but we couldn't do one without the other. I put her on a protocol to eliminate the solvents, which tend to hide in the fat cells—so the protocol involved a far infrared sauna (to release the solvents into her bloodstream), alternating hot and cold (constitutional hydrotherapy) to flush the solvents into her organs of elimination, castor oil packs to help her liver dump into her colon, and colonics to trigger bile dumping and eliminate the solvents from her body entirely. She was to perform this protocol a minimum of three times per week for a minimum of six weeks.

We also did food allergy testing in office, but I knew it would come back with a sensitivity to almost everything. Patricia was concerned there would be nothing left that she could eat.

"We won't eliminate it all," I told her, "just the top offenders."

I also changed the way she dosed her hydrocortisone to three times daily instead of twice daily, and I switched her from Levothyroxine to the natural thyroid, NatureThroid, but at an equivalent dose. Then I gave her a lab requisition form to re-check her thyroid in 6 more weeks.

When Patricia returned three weeks later to review the food allergy results, she told me she was already feeling better: the fatigue had begun to lift just a little, and the rash was mostly gone.

Sure enough, her IgG food allergies were off the charts. The scale goes from 0 to 6, so I took out only the ones in the 5-6 range (which was still a list of about nine foods). I also gave her glutamine to heal up the gut lining, as the food for the small intestine, and probiotics to help her repopulate with the good stuff.

Three weeks later, Patricia returned to follow up on her labs. They showed that her thyroid was actually suppressed, so we lowered her NatureThroid dose. She said her fatigue had improved dramatically, so much so that she had cut her hydrocortisone dose in half on her own. The rash had disappeared completely, and her gut had already responded to treatment (which I told her was unusual—most people don't notice much difference until about week 4 on an allergy elimination protocol).

Three weeks after that, Patricia had stopped her hydrocortisone entirely. She'd gotten busy and stopped doing the detox protocol because she didn't think she needed it anymore. She asked if we could re-check her thyroid again, and we transitioned her to a rotation diet in which she continued to avoid the highest food allergens except very occasionally, and she rotated some of the lower offenders such that she at least was not consuming them daily.

After that, Patricia came in for check-ups from time to time; each time we run lab work, we find we need to lower her thyroid dose a little bit more.

Putting it All Together

In Patricia's case, there was one major obstacle to cure (the solvents—see Chapter 11), and one secondary obstacle (an unhealthy gut, see Chapter 14). As long as those were in the way, nothing else could improve. But as soon as we removed the solvents and healed up her gut so that she could absorb the micronutrients she needed to heal the rest of her (see Chapter 2), then we could taper her off the medications. This was because the underlying need for them had been removed.

Case 3

"I'm no better," Howard told me woefully, fixing me with a pleading expression. "I'm a mess, doc, aren't I?"

This was Howard's fourth visit. He was a sweet man in his seventies, and he'd been to every specialist in the book. Originally he came in with IBS, frequent urination, and insomnia.

"Now, wait a minute," I told him, keeping my finger on the assessment section of his chart note from his third visit. "You told me last time that your gut symptoms had completely resolved!" (We'd put him on a candida protocol. That was all it took.)

"Oh, yes, that is better!" he amended. "But I'm still waking up four times a night to go to the bathroom, and I'm just so tired. I'm such a mess, aren't I?"

I was never quite sure if he was looking for reassurance, or if that was just his refrain. But as usual, I told him, "You're not a mess. We've already gotten your gut better in three visits, and that's been bothering you for years, remember? We'll figure this out too."

Howard had BPH (Benign Prostatic Hypertrophy), but he'd already tried two medications to reduce his prostate inflammation and could not tolerate the side effects. He and I had already attempted Saw Palmetto and Pygeum to reduce the swelling, but it didn't help enough. I'd also hoped the candida protocol might take care of the frequent urination, since that is a common symptom of candida overgrowth—but he still woke too frequently.

"Ok, but remember, you just told me that now

you're only waking four times per night. Last time you told me it was six. It's still too often, but it is improvement!"

"Well, I guess you're right," he concluded doubtfully. "I guess I'm just depressed. My wife tells me I'm too negative. Do you think I'm too negative?"

I smiled. "Focusing on the negative is a habit," I told him, "but there's a way to break it. What I want you to do is to start a gratitude practice. Every day, write down five things that you are grateful for that happened that day. Not generic stuff—really focus on specifics."

"I can do that," he promised me.

We also put him on glycine to attempt to reduce the frequency of his nighttime waking. "I'm pretty sure the insomnia is secondary to the urination issue," I told him.

Howard had told me he was a Christian, so I asked if I could pray with him at the end of the visit. His eyes grew wide.

"Oh, I really must be a lost cause!"

A month later, Howard returned. "I'm still not any better, doc. But I'm trying to be positive… My gut *is* better! We did fix that and I never thought it would improve. Maybe I should just be content with that. If I'm too complicated, you can just tell me to go away and see somebody else…"

"You're not too complicated! We'll get you there," I assured him again. "How often are you going to the bathroom now during the day?"

"About every two hours."

"Ok, that's pretty normal. How often are you waking at night?"

"About three or four times per night."

"That is still a bit of an improvement, but not as much as I'd like," I frowned. I did a search for alternative meds for BPH that he had not yet tried. We found one, and gave it a shot.

We prayed together again, and I urged him to continue his gratitude practice.

Howard cancelled his follow-up, but he sent me email thanking me for all my help. Both the nighttime urination and the insomnia resolved, and he could tolerate this drug with no problems.

Putting it All Together

Howard's obstacles to cure were an unhealthy gut (see Chapter 14), a limiting belief (in this case, "I'm not improving," or "I will never improve"—which then affected his mood and became his reality), and inflammation of his prostate. (Some of this was hormone imbalance, as the earlier treatments worked a bit—see Chapter 17. Unfortunately we never ultimately found a root cause for this, we merely managed the symptom. But as it enabled him to sleep, I was content with that.)

The building blocks Howard required were micronutrients, a side benefit of healing his gut (Chapter 2); sleep (Chapter 5); and peace and a sense of purpose (Chapter 9).

Case 4

Bill immediately struck me as no-nonsense: a businessman in his fifties, he crossed his arms across his thick chest as he sat down.

When I opened with my usual question of "Tell me a little about yourself," he told me, "Well, frankly I'm not sure I believe in naturopathic medicine. My wife made the appointment for me."

"That happens a lot," I nodded and smiled. "So tell me what you've got going on."

"Well, I'm on a lot of medications, and I know I shouldn't be. Maybe you can suggest something natural instead."

I noted from his paperwork that he was on six medications, three for his blood pressure including one diuretic, one for cholesterol, one for sleep, and one antidepressant.

Then he proceeded to list off his chief concerns of high blood pressure, high cholesterol, weight gain, insomnia, and "stress." I asked what "stress" meant.

"Oh, I guess I have a bit of an anger problem," he shrugged.

As he spoke and I typed, I glanced at the first page of his new patient paperwork, where in response to the question, "On a scale of 1 to 10, how committed are you to doing what it takes to improve?" he'd said 6. His self-disclosed diet on the paperwork listed mostly fast or processed foods, and in the "How often do you exercise?" section, his response was 0 hours per week.

"I think we can get your symptoms under control," I told him, "but it's going to require some changes." I launched into a basic healthy eating plan, whole foods based and minimizing sugar, with plenty of veggies. I suggested ways he might restructure his time to create space for exercise, and stress management—including doing things he enjoyed.

"Look, I'm not looking for a lifestyle overhaul," he told me. "I just wanted to get off all the drugs if I can, or at least some of them."

"I'm afraid that's not how that works," I said. "I can't just take you off medications without addressing the reason why they were necessary in the first place. That would be irresponsible of me. Naturopathic philosophy isn't about symptom management; it's about getting rid of the reason why the symptoms are there."

"You can't just give me an herb or something to lower my cholesterol?"

"Well, there are some herbs that will do that," I admitted, "but you're not even well managed on the meds, and most natural substances frankly don't work nearly as well as the drugs do for symptom management. But if you'll make some lifestyle changes now, most likely we can start to wean you off the meds down the line. I get that you don't want a major lifestyle overhaul right now, so I can give you the plan in small steps that don't seem too over-whelming, and then we can add to it a little at a time. But that means it'll probably be awhile before you'll be at the point where we can start to wean you off."

When Bill left, he seemed dissatisfied. I'd been surprised before, but I doubted he'd follow through on the plan. I wondered if I'd even see him again.

Putting it All Together

Bill's obstacle to cure was primarily a limiting belief (see Chapter 18)—in this case, the belief was that he was not in control of or responsible for his health. I couldn't do anything about that without his consent and cooperation.

It was also quite possible that several of his symptoms were side effects of the many meds he was on, or a toxic buildup from pharmaceuticals (Chapter 12). I'd wondered about this particularly with the antidepressant and insomnia, as that is a common side effect.

Had we been able to remove his obstacles, the building blocks he would have needed to heal would have included micronutrients (Chapter 1), macronutrients (Chapter 2), sleep (Chapter 5), exercise (Chapter 6), rest and relaxation (Chapter 7), peace and a sense of purpose (Chapter 9).

I hope you are beginning to see the big picture of naturopathic philosophy, and how identifying and removing obstacles to cure and giving the body what it needs to heal itself can be an art as well as a science.

I invite you to skip to the chapters on those obstacles to cure, and those building blocks that seem most relevant to your own case. Again, you will find the chapters on the most common obstacles in Part 2, and the basic building blocks in Part 1. I'll intersperse shorter patient stories throughout to help illustrate my points, when possible.

Here's to your better health!

Part 2:

What Your Body Needs to

Heal Itself

CHAPTER 1

Building Block #1: Macronutrients

The goal of this chapter is to discuss the three macronutrients: protein, carbohydrates, and fat. You need all of them to be healthy; you just need the good forms of them, and not the crappy, processed forms. At the end of this chapter, you should understand how to tell the difference.

Fat

Contrary to popular belief, **fat is not bad.** You need fat in your diet. For one thing, your brain is almost entirely made of fat, as are the sheaths around your nerve cells. Fat protects your internal organs, it's a great energy source, and it's necessary to absorb your fat soluble vitamins (A, E, D, and K). It's necessary for healthy cell membranes, so that good stuff (nutrients, oxygen, cell signals) can get in, and bad stuff (waste) can get out.

Without enough fat in your diet, you will likely feel fatigued, depressed, and more prone to illness, because many fats are highly antimicrobial.

Unfortunately, the "fat free" craze has led to near elimination of the good fats, instead replacing them with sugar and "bad fats." Here's how to tell the difference between the two.

Quick Chemistry Interlude:

Fats are made up primarily of carbon atoms bonded together. Each carbon can make four bonds. A *saturated fat* is one that is already bonded to as many hydrogens as it can hold.

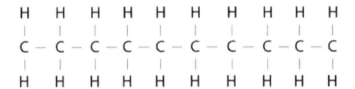

An *unsaturated fat* is one that has space for more hydrogens.

```
H    H    H    H    H    H    H    H    H    H
|    |    |    |    |    |    |    |    |    |
C —  C =  C —  C —  C —  C =  C —  C —  C —  C —
|         |    |         |         |    |    |
H         H    H                   H    H    H
```

Neither of these are inherently bad, but it's mostly the latter that can turn into bad forms of fat. Here's how that happens.

Unhealthy Fats

1) **Trans fats, aka Partially Hydrogenated Oils.** In 1907, Proctor & Gamble devised the process of hydrogenation of plant oils in order to render them solid at room temperatures.[1] *Hydrogenation* means bombarding the unsaturated (liquid) fat with hydrogen ions to make it saturated. But it doesn't work so neatly as that. Instead of a fully saturated backbone, you tend to get trans fats, which have hydrogens on opposite sides of the carbon chain instead of on the same side, like this.

* * *

"Trans" fatty acid

This is bad because these fats won't lay flat against each other, the way natural saturated fats do. If trans fats get into your cell membranes, it means signals don't get in and out of the cells very efficiently. It also means nutrients and oxygen can't get in easily, nor can metabolic waste get out. This matters, because toxic buildup is one of the primary causes for the inflammatory diseases of Western culture (such as diabetes, heart disease, autoimmune conditions, allergies, and cancer).

Trans fats are found in margarine, shortening, processed and fried foods of all kinds.

2) Polyunsaturated vegetable oils. These are commonly used in processed and fast foods, at which point they become trans fats, under conditions of pressure and high heat.

Many vegetable oils are omega 6 essential fatty acids, which are necessary in moderation. The ideal ratio of omega 6 to omega 3 essential fatty acids should be about 4-6:1, in favor of omega 6. But in the Standard American Diet, the ratio is more like

20:1. (Yikes!)

Why this is a problem: if you get just enough omega 6, you'll produce an anti-inflammatory molecule (called a prostaglandin). If you get too much, though, you'll flood the biochemical pathway and produce an inflammatory prostaglandin, which leads to pain—in fact, the inflammatory prostaglandin produced with too much omega 6 is the very chemical suppressed by aspirin.

In other words, *inflammatory pain may be caused by eating too much omega 6 (mostly from vegetable oil and processed foods) and too little omega 3.*

So if you avoid omega 6 polyunsaturated vegetable oils for the most part, chances are you'll end up consuming some here and there by default, and end up at right around the appropriate ratio with omega 3 fatty acids.

Polyunsaturated vegetable oils to stay away from include: canola oil, corn oil, cottonseed oil, safflower and sunflower oil.

Healthy Fats

Saturated Fats. These get a bad rap because too much saturated fat necessarily means too few essential fatty acids (see #3), which leads to inflammation. But if you eat saturated fat in moderation, you reap the benefits, and your body can convert the excess to essential fatty acids if it needs them. Saturated fat makes up 50% of your cell membranes (and healthy cell membranes means good stuff can in, and bad stuff can get out). They are also the preferred food for your heart, they're antimicrobial, they support immune function, they are necessary for your blood to clot and for your lungs to work properly, they are easily absorbed for quick energy, and they are necessary for infant brain development.

What you don't want to do is consume the saturated fat that comes from agriculture industry meats. Animals fed on their natural free-range diets have a 50/50 ratio of saturated fat to essential fatty acids; grain-fed agriculture industry animals' fat is almost 100% saturated. This can lead to inflammation due to the deficiency in essential fatty acids (more on this later in this chapter.)

The saturated fats you should consume are found in coconut oil, avocados, nuts, butter, ghee, palm oil, animal fats (grass fed and/or free range) and eggs (free range).

Monounsaturated Fats. Remember the picture of saturated versus unsaturated fats? Monounsaturated fats have only a single double bond in the chain. These are known to lower inflammatory omega 6, lower cholesterol and blood pressure, and maintain healthy nerve function. The most famous monounsaturated fat is olive oil—just make sure it's "organic" and "extra virgin," as this means it's unprocessed, and therefore still high in antioxidants.

Polyunsaturated Essential Fatty Acids (EFAs): these are the most beneficial type of fat, mostly because it's so probable that you're not eating enough of them. They're anti-inflammatory, they support the mucus lining in your stomach, lower blood pressure and cholesterol, improve insulin sensitivity, decrease allergic responses, keep cell walls healthy, and are necessary for brain development.

EFAs are found in veggie oils (such as flax seed and hemp seed), nut oils (macadamia, peanut), plant oils (pumpkin seed, grape seed, sesame, rice bran, borage, black currant, evening primrose), grass fed meat and dairy, and fish or marine oils.

One more thing before I leave the topic of fats…

A Word On Cholesterol

Cholesterol is not one of the major macronutrients; it's a carrier for fat, essentially. Fat gets stored as triglycerides, and triglycerides get packaged into either HDL (High Density Lipoproteins) or LDL (Low Density Lipoproteins), depending on whether they're headed to your liver to get broken down and used as energy, or whether they're headed from your liver to the rest of you to get stored as fat (respectively).

Despite its reputation for causing heart disease (which is misplaced), adequate levels of cholesterol are quite important, because cholesterol is a precursor for other things you need.

Just like saturated fats and essential fatty acids, **cholesterol is necessary for healthy cell membranes.** If your cell membranes aren't healthy, you won't be able to effectively let nutrients, oxygen, and glucose in, let waste out, or facilitate intracellular communication.

Cholesterol is also the precursor for estrogen, progesterone, testosterone, and all of the hormones produced by your adrenal glands, including DHEA, cortisol, and aldosterone. If you're a man, you definitely want to have plenty of testosterone (more in Chapter 17). If you're a woman, you definitely want to have sufficient estrogen and progesterone, especially if you're peri- or post-menopausal.

Adequate cholesterol is necessary to produce Vitamin D. The active form of it comes from sunlight, of course, but you still have to have enough cholesterol in order to make it. Lack of vitamin D can lead to poor immune function, poor calcium absorption, and depression.

Cholesterol is the precursor for bile, necessary to absorb fat. If you don't have enough bile, then you're going to have trouble with fatty foods, and you won't be able to absorb fat-soluble vitamins either (A, D, E, and K).

Too-high cholesterol is a signal that you have a problem, but it is not the problem itself. Cholesterol functions kind of like a band-aid: levels go up when there's damage to the lining of the blood vessels for some reason. Two of the most common causes of such damage are high sugar intake and smoking. I'll discuss this more in Chapter 10.

My Conclusion on Fat:

Avoid trans fats or high omega 6 fats. Do consume plenty of good fats, including saturated fats from natural, organic sources, monounsaturated and polyunsaturated omega 3 fats.

Also, be sure you're choosing the right fats for the right kinds of cooking. Some of even the healthy fats will go rancid with high heat, forming free radicals, while others are relatively stable. For this reason, you should choose different fat sources depending on your purpose.

• **For high heat cooking,** use animal fats, butter or ghee, coconut oil, or palm oil.

- **For light cooking**, use olive oil, avocado oil, macadamia nut, peanut, sesame, or rice bran oil.
- **For dressings:** use flax, grape seed, hemp, or pumpkin oils.

Protein

All of your cells are made up of proteins. Protein, in turn, is made up of amino acids (twenty of them, to be exact). Your DNA codes for each one of those individual amino acids and, like beads on a chain, your cells assemble the amino acids in sequence such that proteins can be formed. Your body is capable of forming some of those amino acids on its own, but there are others, called essential amino acids, which you have to ingest from your diet (see Table 1). If you don't, you will be malnourished—meaning your body will not be able to perform some of its essential functions.

Table 1

Essential Amino Acids	Conditionally Non-essential	Non-essential Amino Acids
Histidine	Arginine	Alanine
Isoleucine	Asparagine	Aspartate
Leucine	Glutamine	Cysteine
Methionine	Glycine	Glutamate
Phenylalanine	Proline	
Threonine	Serine	
Tryptophan	Tyrosine	
Valine		
Lysine		

The most abundant sources of protein are meat and animal products, such as eggs, cheese, and dairy. Fish and seafood fall under this category too. Vegetarian sources include beans, tofu, nuts, and seeds.

This is a good place to cover the question that generally comes up in this category, and that is this: *aren't vegetarian sources of protein healthier than animal-based sources?*

The China Study was the source of this argument. The most comprehensive study in nutrition ever conducted, it spanned 65 counties in China and resulted in over 8000 statistically significant associations between diet, lifestyle, and disease.[2] They compared the plant-based rural diets in certain parts of China to the Americanized Western diet, which includes high amounts of meat. Not surprisingly, they found that Westernized parts of China experienced far higher incidences of Western diseases of affluence (including cardiovascular disease, diabetes, autoimmune disease, and cancer), compared to those parts of China still consuming their whole food, plant-based fare.

The conclusion was that increased meat intake is responsible for the Western diseases of affluence.

The problem with this reasoning is that correlation does not equal causation. Absolutely, the Western diet stinks, but Western agriculture industry meat products are not the equivalent of the meat that comes from the organic, grass-fed, free-range animals our ancestors have eaten for centuries—long before Western diseases rose to such prominence.

What's So Bad about Agriculture Industry Meat?

Feedlots are designed to make a profit, like any business. The more animals they can raise and slaughter in a given amount of time, the more profit they make. In order to maximize this turnover, however, conditions for the animals are poor… which is bad news, even if you are not an animal activist. Because infection in rampant, dairy cows alone consume about 70% of the nation's antibiotics, contributing to the problem of antibiotic-resistant bacteria.[3]

On top of that, to fatten up the animals for slaughter, they are fed grain (mostly corn) instead of grass. Cow stomachs are not designed to digest corn. This leads to a weakened immune system and increased susceptibility to infection, increasing the need for prophylactic antibiotics (thus speeding development of antibiotic resistant bacteria even more). Also, animals who consume corn instead of grass produce meat whose fat is completely saturated, compared to the 50/50 ratio of saturated to polyunsaturated fats produced by grass-fed animals. Again, some saturated fat is necessary, but in excess it can lead to a relative deficiency of essential fatty acids, leading to inflammation.

If that weren't enough, the corn these animals consume is genetically modified… and the evidence suggests that GMO foods lower the animals' nutrient absorption.[4] When we, in turn, eat the meat from these animals, this lower nutrient content gets passed along to us.

* * *

What's So Good about Organic and Grass-Fed Meat?

Organic, grass-fed animals are allowed to roam free (at least in theory—this isn't well regulated) and consume their natural diet of grass. As a result, not only is the treatment of the animals significantly more humane, but the fat in the meat is about a 50/50 ratio of saturated fats to anti-inflammatory and heart healthy essential fatty acids; the nutrient content of the meat remains intact; and the necessity for antibiotics dramatically declines.

Additionally, adding meat and animal products to your diet provides a much more substantial serving of protein than most plant-based protein sources can provide.

Vegetarian Proteins

If you choose to avoid animal products, the main nutrients you will need to monitor and possibly replace are iron and B12, which are found primarily in meat. The lack of either or both of these can contribute to fatigue, and potentially other deficiency symptoms as well (more on specific nutrient deficiencies in Chapter 2).

If you're a vegetarian, you will need to be vigilant about your protein intake, as you need adequate protein and fats to prevent the blood sugar roller coaster from a diet comprised primarily of carbohydrates, and to keep your gut flora balanced.

Laine was a 25-year old world traveler, who came to me in between trips with constant gas and bloating, brain fog, and fatigue. She was vegan, and proud of her healthy, whole-foods-based diet. However, her diet diary showed that as a result, she consumed mostly grains and fruit, with occasional vegetables. Every now and then she added in nuts or tofu, but inconsistently at best. While she did a great job of choosing nutrient-dense foods, the lack of protein caused the comparatively simple carbs in grains and fruit to hit her bloodstream quickly, feeding the population of candida (a fungal organism) in her gut. As a byproduct, these candida produced gas, and caused her other symptoms.

Once we restricted all simple carbs, killed off the organisms, repopulated with good gut flora, and Laine became vigilant about combining some form of protein with every meal and every snack, her symptoms resolved.

Historically vegetarians relied on soy as a protein staple, but soy has been vilified and thus is falling out of favor. Men avoid it out of fear that it may cause them to develop breast tissue, also known as gynecomastia. Women avoid it out of fear that it may throw their already precarious thyroid numbers out of balance, or that it may increase the risk of hormone-based cancers. I'll address the thyroid and phytoestrogen issues separately.

Phytoestrogens are 100 to 1000 times weaker than the estrogen your body produces naturally. What this means: both types of molecules bind to estrogen receptors the same way a key might fit into a lock—but the resulting effects of this match will be very different. If you have too few natural estrogen molecules in your body, such as in menopause, phytoestrogens will bind to your estrogenic receptors and weakly stimulate them, which may help improve symptoms of too little estrogen. If you have too much estrogen relative to progesterone, however (such as in endometriosis, PMS, some menstrual migraines, etc), then a phytoestrogen will still stimulate that estrogen receptor, but it will do so 100 to 1000 times less than the estrogen molecule that otherwise would have occupied that spot. In other words, phytoestrogens can be either estrogenic *or* anti-estrogenic, depending on which one your body needs.

So I wouldn't worry about soy just because it's a phytoestrogen, unless you have a personal history of an estrogen receptor positive cancer, and you are carefully avoiding *all* estrogenic stimulation.

Maria came to me when she was 48, post-menopause, with fatigue, hot flashes, night sweats, mood swings, and headaches. She'd gotten much worse when her Primary Care Physician prescribed estrogen for her symptoms, and she came to me looking for alternatives. My assessment was that, while her hormones were all quite low, her estrogen was relatively higher than her progesterone levels.

She did not want to take progesterone, having been a bit "snake-bit" with hormones already. So instead I put her on a diet eliminating sugar, white carbohydrates, and caffeine, increasing cruciferous veggies, and increasing her non-GMO soy intake. This turned out to be all she needed: a regular dose of soy balanced her hormones well enough that her symptoms disappeared.

The connection between soy and thyroid suppression has nothing to do with its status as a phytoestrogen. Several other foods considered to be thyroid suppressants (aka *goitrogens*) include millet, peanuts, radishes, turnips, and raw cruciferous veggies (such as cauliflower, brussels sprouts, and broccoli). These are very healthy foods overall, and it would be a mistake to completely avoid them. Goitrogens are only a problem for thyroid function if you're already iodine deficient. Iodine is one of the minerals necessary for the formation of thyroid hormone, and goitrogens compete with thyroid hormone for iodine. So as long as your iodine status is not a problem, you need not avoid these foods—including soy. Even if you *are* iodine deficient (which isn't uncommon—I run blood tests for this all the time), fermenting, cooking, or steaming these goitrogens renders them safe for consumption. Fermented soy products include natto, miso, soy sauce, and tempeh.

However (and this is a big however), soy is one of the foods that is most commonly genetically modified—we're talking 94% of the soy in the U.S. It still isn't absolutely clear what sorts of ramifications genetic modification may have on health, but because there is plenty of evidence to suggest there might be a problem, I choose to play it safe and avoid GMO soy (more on this in chapter 10).

The other major plant-based protein source, beans, contain carbohydrates that are difficult to break down, which can contribute to gas and bloating. For this reason, my vegetarian and vegan patients whose guts are not especially robust tend to have a harder time consuming adequate protein.

High Protein Fad Diets

You don't want to emphasize protein too much either, contrary to such fad diets as South Beach, Atkins, and Bernstein. While these diets will lower cholesterol, triglycerides, insulin resistance, and weight, too *much* protein over a period of time can lead to kidney damage, weight loss, and (depending on the type of protein consumed) high saturated fat relative to essential fatty acids. It can also set you up for nutrient deficiencies if your primary source of nutrition is meat. Also, your body runs on glucose from carbohydrates, not protein—so although it is possible for your body to turn protein into energy, it's not nearly as efficient, so you may feel exhausted. And finally, the lack of fiber inherent in high protein diets may lead to constipation.

Jeff came to me with bloating and constipation with almost any carbohydrate he put into his mouth. He'd learned to deal with this by eating almost exclusively protein. I frowned when I saw this, and asked to see his most recent blood work to check his kidneys. He told me he hadn't brought it, but that doctors in the past had told him he had kidney problems. He also said he could not drink enough water to stay hydrated.

I sent him home with a stool culture, suspecting candida and possibly some other dysbiotic organism causing the symptoms, and also recommended electrolytes and the amino acid taurine to assist with his absorption of fluids. While we waited for the results, I recommended that he restrict protein to no more than 30% of his diet, and add in fish oil for further kidney protection.

Jeff was positive for candida, and also two other pathogenic bacteria. At the next visit he told me he did feel that he was hydrating much better. I put him on a diet and supplement protocol for six weeks, and sent him home with a requisition to re-check his kidneys. Six weeks later, his bloating and constipation with carbs was resolved, and kidney function had returned to normal on lab work.

My Conclusion on Protein:

For most healthy patients, I encourage organic or free-range animal protein consumption as part of a balanced, whole-foods diet, except for those who abstain for religious or ethical reasons. There are certain conditions which do require avoiding animal proteins for a period of time, though, such as gallstones.

And I will say this: If your choice is between whole food vegetarianism or veganism and the Standard American Diet, there's no doubt that the former is healthier!

Carbohydrates ("Carbs")

As previously mentioned, carbohydrates are the macronutrient most efficiently turned into glucose, which is your body's primary fuel source. The more complex the carbohydrates are (i.e. the bigger the molecule), the more work your body has to do in order to release its energy potential. Another way to say this is that complex carbs have a lower glycemic index.

The glycemic index is a measure of how quickly a particular food turns to sugar in the body. Glucose is assigned a glycemic index of 100, and everything else is assigned a number relative to that. At the top of the glycemic index list are all things white, especially processed white flour (including white bread, pancakes, and pastries), most processed white grains (including white rice, instant oatmeal, popcorn, and most cereals), and white potatoes, especially potato products (including french fries, potato chips, and instant mashed potatoes). The most complex carbohydrates, those with the lowest glycemic index, are generally vegetables (starchy ones excepted), followed by fruit and whole grains.

Sugar tastes good to us because it's a source of quick energy, which historically was a lot more scarce than it is today. It can get converted into ATP, the currency your body uses for energy, very quickly. But your blood can only accommodate a few tablespoons of sugar at a time.

Picture table sugar—it's granular and it has relatively rough edges. If you have too much sugar in your bloodstream over a period of time, those rough edges nick the walls of your blood vessels and cause damage. When that happens, your body has to patch up the damage with a "band-aid," so that it can heal. The "band-aid" is called LDL (aka "bad" cholesterol). The more extensive the damage, the more cholesterol you need to form an adequate band-aid. But with continued high intake of sugar, over time that LDL plug gets bigger and bigger. Eventually it may impede blood flow, or the plug can become unstable and break off, traveling to some other part of the body until it encounters a blood vessel too small to accommodate it. (This is cardiovascular disease—and it can lead to heart attacks and strokes.) **Cardiovascular disease is problem #1 with too much sugar.** (Note that the LDL was *not* the culprit —it only showed up to try to fix the problem!)

So your body tries to get rid of excess sugar from the bloodstream in order to minimize this process. Sugar has to get inside the cells in order to get out of the blood. Sugar can't just rush into the cells directly though—it has to have the "key" to get in. The key is insulin, and it gets produced from the pancreas in response to high sugar in the bloodstream. This works great for awhile… but problems come in when this cycle is repeated too often, too long. Like a drug addict needing a bigger dose to achieve the same high, the body will start to require more and more insulin to keep up with your sugar intake. Eventually, the pancreas can't keep up with the demand. This leads to **Insulin Resistance and Diabetes, problem #2 with too much sugar.**

Once the sugar gets inside the cells, it can't be stored in its present form—it has to be converted from "quick" energy into "potential" energy—aka fat (or more precisely, triglycerides.) So sugar also leads to obesity. **Obesity is problem #3 with too much**

sugar.

There are even more potential issues that this. But for now, suffice it to say that too much sugar is no small part of the epidemic of obesity, diabetes, and cardiovascular disease in this nation. The average American consumes about 156 pounds of it per year![5]

My Conclusions on Carbohydrates

The best carbs are veggies, hands down. They are super nutrient dense, and full of fiber that will help to keep your gut healthy and eliminate toxins. A healthy diet will also include 100% whole (i.e. unprocessed) grains and a variety of different types of fruits—the more colorful the better.

You don't want a diet that's primarily complex carbs to the exclusion of adequate fat and protein, though. High carb fad diets such as Ornish, Pritikin, McDougall, and Swank Diets will lead to lower cholesterol and triglycerides, weight loss, lower cardiovascular and cancer risk, and a healthier gut due to the high fiber. However, they can set you up for deficiencies in essential fatty acids (since those are fat), and in fat-soluble vitamins (A, D, E, and K). Some people also feel inordinately hungry on a high carb diet, and potentially hypoglycemic.

Do minimize sugar and simple carbs as much as you can. Make them an occasional treat, rather than a dietary staple.

To Recap: How, Then, Should You Eat?

• Keep grains to a minimum. Healthy grains to choose include quinoa, brown or wild rice,
• sprouted wheat, corn, millet, spelt, and kamut.
• Eat as many vegetables, in as many different colors, as possible.
• Try and limit fruit to 1-2 times per day. Fruit is nutritious but high in sugar. The best fruits to choose are berries, as they are lower on the glycemic scale than other fruits, and quite high in antioxidants.
• Add some form of protein to every meal, including every snack. If you eat animal products, choose organic if you can afford it, or free range; avoid purchasing agriculture industry animal products. Other healthy proteins include tofu (non-GMO of course), nuts and nut butters, beans and hummus, yogurt (especially Greek), and fish (go for Alaskan or Pacific and wild caught, never farm raised). Quinoa is also high in protein, for a grain.
• Cook with healthy fats, appropriate to the heat setting you're using.

• Read labels: avoid added sugar and ingredients you don't recognize (more on this in Part 2). Lists should consist of whole foods primarily.

CHAPTER 2

Building Block #2: Micronutrients

The other part of the nutritional equation are the micronutrients that your body needs.

A *nutrient* is a catch-all term for any substance that provides the building blocks for replenishment of an organism (so it includes vitamins, minerals, essential fatty acids, essential amino acids, and also macronutrients, such as carbs, protein, and fats).

Vitamins and *minerals* (those nutrients normally found in a multivitamin) are distinct from macronutrients in that they don't provide energy; rather, they help the body carry out some of its vital functions (hence the prefix *vita-*, as in vitality). A vitamin is a more complex molecule, while a mineral is a single element in the periodic table (though it's almost always bound to something else for the purpose of delivery, and so forms a compound. What it's bound to makes a difference in terms of absorbability.)

Once upon a time, we could get all of these nutrients straight from our diets. Unfortunately for most of us, that's no longer true. Here's why.

Soil Requirements for Healthy Plants

Plants need essential nutrients from soil just like you need them from your food—some in large amounts, and some in trace amounts. Primary nutrients for plants include nitrogen, phosphorus and potassium. If you look at commercial fertilizer bags, the label will usually say N-P-K, representing these major nutritional requirements.

Intermediate nutrient requirements are sulfur, magnesium, and calcium.

Micronutrients include boron, copper, iron, chloride, manganese, molybdenum, zinc, cobalt, and nickel.

Too little of any one of them can affect the health of the plant, and its nutrient value to its consumers.

What Affects Nutrient Content in Soil

A few variables affect this. One is texture: basically the more the soil holds on to water (moisture and stickiness), the more it will hold on to nutrients as well. Sand obviously doesn't grow much (hence the barren deserts), while clay and organic soil does.

Another is pH. Just like our bodies have to maintain the right pH for life, so soil has to stay in the right pH range (6.0-6.5) to release both macro and micronutrients from the soil to the plants. Otherwise these nutrients will be bound up and unavailable. The right pH will also allow growth of microbe populations that help to convert the nutrients nitrogen and sulfur into usable forms for the plant. (By the way, you need plenty of microbes to help you with your digestion too!)

Fertilizer: What To Do When Soil is Suboptimal

If your soil lacks either the nutrients or the pH for growth (or both), you have to fertilize. This is where the difference between commercial and organic farming comes in.

Commercial fertilizers are processed to adjust the pH rapidly and provide a walloping dose of synthetic nutrients, and they are great for giving a jump-start to very depleted soil. These nutrients are mined, chemically processed, and delivered to the soil in salt form (much like our table salt, made from rock salt). These salts release their nutrients to the soil quickly and easily when they come in contact with water.

The problem is, these fertilizers add primarily macronutrients for the plant's use, but they don't help the soil to cultivate those necessary micronutrients. (Think of it like a human subsisting entirely on fast food. You may be getting all three of the major macronutrients: carbs, protein, and fat, but you're still malnourished, and it'll catch up with you eventually.) In the same way, this means that even though the plants may grow rapidly (just like you would on a fast food diet!), over time the soil gets depleted of its micronutrients. Maybe the first generation of plants grown in that soil will have all they need, but eventually those micronutrients get consumed and the soil will thus become unhealthy. This means future generations will lack those micronutrients necessary for the health of the plants, and they'll pass these deficiencies on to you.

If that weren't enough, sickly plants also tend to become targets for pests, which makes pesticides increasingly necessary (many of which are toxic to humans. As a side note on this: notice that the healthier the soil, the more easily they repel pests on their own, just like healthy humans will require far less outside assistance to prevent illness. Antibiotics, like pesticides, will work in a pinch... but they aren't dealing with the underlying issue, which is why the susceptibility exists in the first place.)

Genetically modified foods (GMO) try to get around the pest issue by adding pesticides directly to the genetic code of the plants… but among other potential problems, evidence demonstrates that GMO foods bind micronutrients such as manganese, zinc, and iron. (Not only is the soil deficient in them, but now what is there isn't available either.) This means sickly plants, sickly animals who eat the plants (since many commercial farming animals are fed from GMO corn or soy), and sickly people who eat those animals. Again, more on this in Chapter 10.

Organic Foods:

Organic fertilizers are created from "natural" substances, rather than in a chemistry lab. These include things like compost, animal manure or guano, blood meal (from powdered blood), fish meal (from ground up fish), bone meal (what it sounds like), and that sort of thing. (So if you think about it… organic plants are sort of carnivorous!)

Because these nutrients are bound up in complex molecules, though, it takes time for soil organisms to decompose the organic fertilizers enough to release the key nutrients into the soil. Really depleted soil will appear to respond much faster to synthetics for this reason, but that approach doesn't aid the health of the soil and the plants in the long run. It's much better to build up the soil with compost, and then fertilize it with organic materials containing all the necessary micronutrients.

Because of this, organic foods are more nutrient dense than their commercial counterparts.[1] If you eat only organic foods (or better yet, if you live on a farm and grow your own), you may be one of the lucky few in our society who don't need to supplement with additional micronutrients.

Eating 100% organic is pretty pricey and not possible for most of us, though. Realistically speaking, because our food is nowhere near as nutrient dense as it used to be, most of us should be on a good, absorbable multivitamin to maintain health.

I look for three main things to determine whether a multi is good or not. First, it should have chelated mineral forms (i.e. look at the magnesium and the calcium and etc: they should be complexed with glycinate or citrate or orotate or taurate, or other chelated forms—but not oxide or sulfate, as these are not absorbable.) Second, dosing recommendations should be multiple times daily. That doesn't mean you have to actually take it multiple times daily, it just means the manufacturer is aware that some of the vitamins are water-soluble, and therefore to maintain a sustained level throughout the day, you should take it more than once. And third, with the exception of whole-foods based vitamins, which are often tablets, you should choose capsules over tablets (particularly if you are older or have low stomach acid). This is because tablets are harder for your gut to break down.

Essential Fatty Acids

These are another supplement that almost everyone should take. They're called *essential* because your body can't synthesize them on its own—you have to ingest them from your diet. And unfortunately, as mentioned in the last chapter, the Standard American Diet has precious few of them. Across the population, average dietary intake of EFAs in North America tends to be around 100 mg per day, whereas healthy individuals should get around 500 mg of EFAs daily.

In With the Good, Out With the Bad

Probably the most important reason why everyone needs EFAs is because they are a critical component to maintaining healthy cell walls.

Historically the "brain" of the cell was considered to be its nucleus, and cell walls were considered to be the "skin." But if you remove the nucleus from a cell, it can still function just fine—it just can't reproduce (implying that the nucleus is more like the cell's reproductive organ than its brain.) But if you remove the cell's membrane, the cell dies immediately. The membrane, therefore, is even more important than the cell's nucleus!

Cell membranes are like gates, and the receptors dotted along the membrane are like gatekeepers. These receptors require a certain "password" in order to open and let a particular substance inside the cell —not just anybody gets in. But the "gate" has to be fluid enough to allow the gatekeepers to do their jobs properly, and also to let out the internal waste left over from cellular processes.

EFAs keep the gate fluid, letting the "good" stuff in and the "bad" stuff out. This is true for every cell in your body. Healthy gates will let in nutrients and oxygen (critical for life!), let in glucose for energy (limiting insulin resistance), let in neurotransmitters in brain cells (improving mood disorders), and maintain proper nerve conduction (treating neuropathy symptoms).

Letting the trash "out" is universally important too, since toxic buildup is one of the primary causes for the inflammatory diseases of Western culture, such as diabetes, heart disease, autoimmune conditions, allergies, and cancer. Also, as mentioned in Chapter 1, EFAs are highly anti-inflammatory.

Fish oil, krill oil, or any other good EFA is comprised of EPA and DHA, which are both in the omega 3 pathway. Taking fish oil daily helps to balance out the ratio of omega 6 to omega 3.

Choosing an EFA

I prefer fish oil to flax seed oil only because the EPA content is higher in fish oil. But I still like flax seed oil, especially for vegans or vegetarians who don't eat fish.

Krill oil is a fine alternative to fish oil, it's just more expensive.

Cod liver oil has not just EFAs, but also Vitamins A and D, which is great for immune support. Depending on the brand, you might have a lower amount of EFAs than pure fish oil, but this isn't universally true.

A word of caution on fish oil: If it smells "fishy" then it's likely rancid, and rancid fish oil actually becomes a pro-oxidant, rather than an antioxidant. Don't let it go beyond its expiration date.

Choose one that says "Pharmaceutical Grade" on

the bottle—this means it's got a much higher percentage of actual omega 3 in the capsule (compared to fillers, like fish fat).

I'd also be careful about purchasing fish oil from a regular pharmacy or a box store. In the case of fish oil, quality matters, because fish is so toxic these days. If you buy cheap fish oil, they probably got it from cheap fish—which was most likely farmed or Atlantic, both of which are chock-full of heavy metals.

Electrolytes

Another class of trace nutrients we all need for life are *electrolytes.*

The word electrolyte generally refers to the largest concentration of charged particles within the human body. The biggest two are sodium (Na^+) and chloride (Cl^-), which, when you put them together, make up the bulk of our salt. These charged particles are critical for your physiology: all of the cells in your body do their work based on the gradient, or separation, of positive and negative charges (kind of like a battery).

This means you have to have the proper balance of electrolytes for life.

Fortunately, your body already has a pretty awesome buffer system built in to maintain these concentrations even when you sweat a little too much, or drink too much reverse osmosis water (more on this in Chapter 4), get dehydrated, or eat a whole bunch of refined crappy salt or processed food high in pure sodium, rather than healthy sea salt (more on this below).

The brunt of this effort to maintain your electrolyte balance falls on your kidneys. You've got to help them out, though—otherwise you'll be setting yourself up for kidney stones and osteoporosis (more on this in Chapter 10). When dehydrated, it's important that you rehydrate not just with pure water, but also with a balance of electrolytes. This is why most sport drinks also contain electrolytes for rehydration, and why it's a good idea to use Pedialyte or a similar product when rehydrating after a bout of acute diarrhea or vomiting.

For general maintenance, though, it's also important to help your kidneys out by taking in a good balance of electrolytes. Don't way overdo the sodium (which is very high in processed foods), but don't skip the salt altogether either. Just make sure you choose the good stuff.

What's In Natural (Sea) Salt

Historically, naturally occurring salt was the only salt available for use. This salt comes from the sea, or from other water sources (such as the Himalayas—hence the popular pink Himalayan salt). This salt contains not just sodium chloride (only around 84% actually), but also a number of other trace minerals. The precise balance of minerals depends on where the salt was harvested from, but generally they include a combination of silicon and phosphorus (both necessary for calcium uptake into bones), vanadium (which helps with blood sugar control), magnesium (a very common deficiency), calcium, and potassium.

How Table Salt is Made

By contrast, most of the salt on American tables starts out as rock salt. It's got a bunch of inedible impurities in it, so it has to be heated in a kiln to 1200 degrees F, changing its chemical structure to sodium chloride (NaCl—processed salt is about 98% this). Then they add anti-caking agents (such as toxic ferrocyanide and aluminosilicate), and in places where there isn't fluorine added to the water, they'll add fluoride to the salt, plus a little potassium iodide (added because we're not getting enough iodine in our diets).

As a general rule, you should avoid any highly

processed substance that masquerades as food. In this case, though, by choosing sea salt, you'll also get a good source of other electrolytes and minerals, which will assist your kidneys in maintaining optimum health.

Antioxidants

We know that oxidative stress is a mediating factor in heart disease, diabetes, cancer, Alzheimer's disease, and chronic inflammatory diseases, and it is postulated to be a major contributor to cellular aging as well. Antioxidants neutralize the free radicals (unpaired electrons that is) that cause oxidative stress. Many nutrients are considered to be antioxidants, but most important are those found throughout the body (called "endogenous"), and those that are capable of regenerating other antioxidants. To protect yourself against the oxidative damage rampant in our modern world, find a complex that contains NAC (N-Acetyl Cysteine), ALA (Alpha Lipoic Acid), and/or CoQ10. There are also specific antioxidants which may be important for a given condition, but it's best to check with your naturopathic doctor which ones are right for you.

Probiotics

Your gut, we are realizing more and more, is the gateway not just to pathogenic illnesses, but also to noninfectious gut disorders like allergies and autoimmunity. It's also the key to protecting against these ailments (more on this in Chapter 3).

Although it may seem unnatural to supplement with microorganisms, people once consumed a much higher volume of fermented foods (and therefore of probiotics) than they do today. Look for a probiotic with 20 billion organisms at about a 50/50 ratio of Lactobacillus and Bifidobacterium, as these are the organisms that make up the majority of the Western culture gut flora, at about that ratio.

Individual Micronutrient Deficiencies

These basic supplement recommendations presuppose an otherwise healthy body. In some cases, though, people need more of a particular nutrient to correct a problem. In general, do not supplement an individual vitamin or mineral without the advice of a nutritionist or naturopathic physician, because overdose or imbalance is possible for some of them, and also because some of these symptoms may be indicative of an underlying condition that you might mask with supplementation.

That said, here's a quick "review of systems," pointing out common issues that may indicate a nutrient deficiency.

Your nails can tell you a lot about potential deficiencies. Ridges, white spots, or hang nails often indicate a zinc deficiency. Soft or brittle nails may indicate a magnesium deficiency.

Hair loss can be a lot of things (more on this in Chapter 16), but biotin, zinc, or iron deficiency are possible causes.

Usually **skin problems** involve the gut and/or the liver, and there are often food intolerances involved (see chapter 14). That said, it may also indicate the following deficiencies:

• Dermatitis (inflamed skin): related to deficiency in Vitamins B2, B3, B6, C, E, A, zinc, and biotin

• Follicular Hyperkeratosis (plugged pores on the backs of the arms): Vitamin A or Essential Fatty Acid deficiency

• Seborrheic Dermatitis (flaky, oily skin): could be a biotin deficiency

• Eczema: potentially Vitamin B2 or Vitamin E deficiency.

• Psoriasis: associated with low Vitamin A, D, E, C, and zinc.

• Acne Vulgaris: associated with deficiency in

Vitamins A, B5, B6, E, and zinc
• Acne Rosacea: associated with deficiency in Vitamins C and B2

Night blindness may indicate vitamin A deficiencies. Dark circles under the eyes, sometimes called "allergic shiners," are often a sign of food intolerance.

Frequent nose bleeds may be a folate or Vitamin B12 deficiency, Vitamin K deficiency, or a lack of antioxidants. Get this worked up if it's frequent.

Issues in your mouth often are B vitamin deficiencies. Specifically:
• Swollen or fissured tongue: may be iron deficiency, or lack of vitamins B2, B3, B6, or B12
• Cracked, peeling lips or edges of the mouth: may be a vitamin B2 deficiency
• Bleeding gums: vitamin C deficiency
• Gum disease: folic acid, CoQ10, or Vitamin C deficiency
• Loss of taste: may be a B12 or zinc deficiency
• Canker sores: may be a B12 or folate deficiency

Tinnitus (ringing in the ears) may be caused by a lot of things, but could be a Vitamin B3, B12 or Vitamin E deficiency. Get this worked up.

Frequent soreness or muscle spasms may be a

magnesium deficiency or an electrolyte imbalance. Along those lines, Restless Leg Syndrome may be caused by a number of things, but can be an electrolyte imbalance, or deficiency in iron, calcium, Vitamin E or folate.

Magnesium Deficiency

Magnesium gets its own section because it's really important, and it's a common deficiency. It is a cofactor for about 300 reactions in your body (meaning it's required for the reaction to proceed). These reactions include making, transporting, and using energy, making DNA and proteins, controlling nerve signals, relaxing muscles, and responding adequately to stress.

Reasons You Might Be Low

You might not be eating enough of the foods that contain magnesium. Magnesium is found in whole grains, nuts, beans, green leafy veggies, fish, and (clean) meat.

Even if you're consuming plenty of these foods, a bunch of pharmaceuticals also block the absorption of magnesium or increase its excretion, including laxatives, diuretics, proton pump inhibitors (like

Nexium), antibiotics, colchicine, and corticosteroids (like prednisone. More on this in Chapter 12).

You can also deplete magnesium by consuming too much alcohol or too many phosphates (from soda —more in Chapter 10).

If you have a hard time absorbing nutrients in general (a malabsorption syndrome, such as Crohn's, celiac sprue, or enteritis, see Chapter 14), then you are likely to be deficient in magnesium also.

You might be deficient if you have Type 2 Diabetes, especially if it isn't well controlled, because high blood sugar leads to increased urination, and like all electrolytes, magnesium reabsorption happens in the kidneys.

How You Know If You're Low

The test for magnesium in your bloodstream (serum magnesium) isn't reliable, because most magnesium stays inside your cells and your bones. Red blood cell (RBC) magnesium is a better test, therefore, because that's testing the magnesium concentration inside the red blood cells.

However, often clinical signs and symptoms, combined with knowledge of one of the five causes listed above is the best way to determine deficiency. Low magnesium can lead to problems with memory and concentration, depression and apathy, emotional lability (you get upset easily), irritability, nervousness, and anxiety, insomnia, constipation, migraines, PMS and cramping, fibromyalgia and muscle pain, fatigue, and ADHD.

Micronutrients Matter

Your body is designed to crave micronutrients as well as macronutrients. You can't give it calories without vitamins and minerals, because the body will still tell you it wants more. It thinks you're starving it if you aren't taking in the former as well.

The Take-Home Message:

•   If organic food is available and affordable, buy it. When organic isn't available or affordable, at least go for whole foods.
•   Get on a good, absorbable multivitamin.
•   Start taking a pharmaceutical grade fish oil or other essential fatty acid.
•   Get yourself on a probiotic (more on this in the next chapter).
•   Consider testing for other nutrient deficiencies and supplementing appropriately.

CHAPTER 3

Building Block #3: A Healthy Gut

Consuming the appropriate balance of macronutrients and micronutrients is of course an absolute essential of health: you have to have the necessary building blocks for repair to occur. But even if you are feeding your body adequate building blocks, it's equally important that you're able to absorb them. This is where your gut comes in.

Digestion In A Nutshell (aka Bowel Transit)

All of the various components of digestion have to work together in order for assimilation of nutrients to happen.

You chew your food, and the enzymes your saliva begin to break down the simple carbs you consume, turning them into glucose. You swallow, and the food travels from your throat (aka pharynx) to your esophagus.

The function of your esophagus is to connect your throat to your stomach, but it's also a muscle, pushing your food downward in rhythmic waves called *peristalsis*.

The esophagus opens into the stomach via the esophageal sphincter. The sphincter is coordinated with the peristaltic waves, opening in response to the waves, and closing in response to the low pH of the stomach acid below it.

Your stomach processes the food bolus you've just swallowed, and the hydrochloric acid breaks down your food into bits for the next stages of the digestive process. Hydrochloric acid is especially necessary for breaking down protein; too little and later stages of digestion won't be able to assimilate nutrients that are still trapped in their organic material, leading to malabsorption. Also, if those bits of food can't go through later stages of digestion, the bacteria in your intestines will break it down for you, leading to gas and bloating.

Your stomach dumps food into your small intestine, where peristalsis continues. Your gut can only absorb simple molecules, so the first part of your small intestine, called the duodenum, receives digestive enzymes from the pancreas to further break down protein, carbs, and fat. Think of enzymes like pairs of scissors that cut bigger molecules into smaller pieces. There's a different pair of scissors, or different enzymes, for different classes of food.

The duodenum also receives bile from your gall bladder (or directly from your liver if your gall bladder has been removed) to emulsify fat and allow its absorption. Bile works on fat the way soap works on dirt. Most toxins from solvents are fat-soluble, so if these have entered your digestive tract, the bile will sweep these up too.

Beneficial bacteria, or probiotics, gobble up whatever's still not simple enough for your body to absorb, and they leave behind lactic acid as a byproduct. This process is called fermentation. A little chemistry digression here: fermentation happens in the absence of oxygen, and it's the conversion of carbohydrates (sugar) to alcohol or lactic acid, and carbon dioxide (CO_2). Lactic acid and/or alcohol act as a natural preservative, because bad bacteria cannot survive in an acidic environment—they keep the "bad" bacteria and yeast in check. They also break down antinutrients (called phytobiotics) that that block the body's ability to absorb vitamins and minerals.

Actual absorption of nutrients occurs mostly in the second and third part of the small intestine (called the jejunum and the ileum). The ileum is also the site of absorption of Intrinsic Factor, which is bound to Vitamin B12. Nutrients from the small intestine get absorbed into the bloodstream, and the blood then goes to the liver to get filtered for any toxins you might have picked up from your food (such as, say, a preservative with a twenty-syllable name).

After extracting all the good stuff, the ileum, the last part of the small intestine, then dumps whatever's left over into the colon. The colon consists of the cecum (the connection between the ileum and the rest of the colon), and then the ascending, transverse, and descending colon, which are what they sound like. The descending colon turns into the sigmoid colon, so named because it's shaped like an S, and it empties into the rectum. Peristalsis continues throughout the colon, pushing waste downward for elimination. The colon also reabsorbs water from the stool, so that it is neither too watery nor too dry.

The rectum is about eight inches long, and acts as a storage reservoir for stool. When it becomes full, the brain tells you that it's time to have a bowel movement (or to release gas, left over from the fermentation process above). The rectum is connected to the anal sphincter, part of the muscles of the pelvic floor. These are voluntary muscles that relax when we get to a toilet.

Ideally this whole process takes about 24 hours.

The Essential Role of Your Microbiome

First, let's define our terms: your *microbiome* is the collective term for all the bacteria that populate your gut—all 100 trillion of them. Even though your microbiome is not technically "you," it's so important to your body's function that it's been characterized as another organ.

Your microbiome acts like an army, protecting you against foreign invaders (pathogenic bacteria, parasites, etc). It also helps to educate your immune system about the difference between friend and foe, making it very important to mitigate against and prevent allergies and autoimmunity. It also helps you break down your food. You know how raw cruciferous veggies and certain kinds of beans can make you gassy? If you had the right balance of bacteria in your microbiome, recent studies show, you wouldn't have that problem. You don't have those bacteria because you just don't need them often enough, relative to other cultures replete with fiber. (Just like with everything else—use it or lose it.)

Different Diets Require Different Organisms

Three studies[1, 2, 3] compare indigenous diets (consisting primarily of veggies, tubers, legumes, and high-fiber grains) to Western diets (consisting primarily of high animal fats—agriculture industry fat, that is—sugar, processed foods, and low fiber).

What they found: first, the distribution of bacteria that make up the microbiome differs, based upon dietary consumption. Hunter-gatherers require more organisms to help break down otherwise undigestible polysaccharides (complex carbs), whereas Western subjects don't eat enough polysaccharides for this to matter. At least that's the assumption.

Second, Western populations have a very high proportion of bifidobacillus in their microbiome, whereas the indigenous populations studied so far have none at all. Bifidobacillus comprises a chunk of the microbiome of nursing infants in all cultures, however—the assumption is that bifidobacillus is correlated with consumption of milk. Cultures that do not consume milk beyond infancy (and most don't) wouldn't require this organism to help break it down into adulthood.

Third, indigenous cultures have a much greater

biodiversity in their microbiomes than do Westerners. This may be due to the lack of diversity in our diets, causing the microbiome to respond by becoming similarly narrow. Another possibility is the overwhelming use of antibiotics, not only among ourselves for minor ailments, but also in the agricultural industry. Once a relatively minor population of gut flora gets wiped out, it won't be able to rebound —as far as our little ecosystem is concerned, it's extinct.

Indigenous Diets = Greater Biodiversity

Turns out the indigenous populations tested had not just greater biodiversity, but also significantly more short-chain fatty acids (SCFA), which are produced by the microflora, than the Western populations. SCFA are the food for the large intestine, allowing it to repair itself.

Your gut, we are realizing more and more, is the gateway not just to pathogenic illnesses, but also to noninfectious gut disorders like allergies and autoimmunity (see Chapter 15). It's also the key to protecting against these ailments.

Healthy Digestion

In Chapter 14, I'll deal more with all the various things that can go wrong in the digestive process, and what to do about them. For now, let's assume digestion is already healthy. Here's how to keep it that way.

1) Make sure you're getting appropriate nutrients.

Eating processed crap can cause a number of issues, but one of them is nutrient deficiency (see Chapter 2)—since processing often involves stripping foods of their nutrients. For example, processed grains typically have been stripped of the fiber and nutrients in the hull, and are left with nothing more than the "white" carbohydrate and the protein (gluten, if it's a gluten-containing grain). Both macronutrients and micronutrients are necessary for your body to function appropriately, and (for the most part) you can only get them by swallowing them.

2) Consume plenty of raw foods.

A food is considered "raw" if it is not heated above 120 degrees, and includes raw milk (unpasteurized and non-homogenized), raw honey, raw cocoa, and raw fruits and veggies, as well as fermented foods such as raw cheese, raw yogurt, raw kefir, sourdough bread, sauerkraut, pickles, wine, fermented beets and carrots, and fermented apple cider. (Note that I am not talking about raw meat here!) Raw foods naturally contain enzymes, probiotics, vitamins, and minerals—which means they actually help you to digest them. But food processing (for example, pasteurization, or even cooking,) tends to destroy these things. Pasteurization involves heating foods to high temperatures in order to kill off bad bacteria. The problem is, in the process, all of the naturally occurring enzymes are destroyed, as well as all of the good bacteria, and a good percentage of the vitamins and minerals.

Therefore, the healthy individual whose gut can handle the extra fiber should shoot for around 50-80% raw food. Not only are raw foods more nutrient-dense, but they'll also take some of the strain off of your digestive system.

3) If organic food is available and affordable, buy it.

As mentioned in the micronutrient section, foods grown in organic soil have a full complement of micronutrients, not just their major macronutrients (which, to them, are nitrogen, potassium, and phosphorus). This means not only will they pass their mineral richness on to you—but because they are healthy themselves, they don't require pesticides and for the most part are grown without them. (This means fewer unrecognizable chemicals for your liver to detoxify—more on this in Chapter 10.) And in the case of the agriculture industry meat products, it means greater nutrient density, less indirect antibiotic or hormone exposure, and far more essential fatty acids, leading to less inflammation.

4) Take your probiotics.

Once again, friendly bacteria protect you against bad bacteria, secrete acid to help you absorb nutrients, and break down any larger food particles that your hydrochloric acid, bile, and enzymes might have missed. Once upon a time, before modern preservation techniques, fermented condiments played a central role in our meals. These helped to replenish friendly bacteria on a regular basis. Back then, we also weren't using over-the-counter acid-blocking medications (PPIs and H2 blockers), nor were we feeding antibiotics to the animals we ate on a regular basis—so the good bacteria we do have weren't nearly so in jeopardy as they are now. If you're one of the very few that have not exposed yourself to medications that alter your gut ecology, you might be able to get away with going back on a diet incorporating regular fermented foods instead of taking a probiotic. For the rest of us, a regular probiotic is essential.

5) Drink half your body weight in ounces daily.

One really common, obvious cause for constipation is simply dehydration. You should drink more than half your body weight in ounces if you live in a dry climate, or if you sweat regularly.

6) Exercise.

Another super common cause for constipation is a sedentary lifestyle. When you exercise, the peristalsis in your gut responds. Eventually you'll also increase your metabolism, which will translate to a quicker bowel transit time, too.

CHAPTER 4

Building Block #4: Water, Fresh Air, and Sunlight

Picture a dim, musty room, with the window all boarded up and the counters and walls covered with dirt and grime. Would you be surprised if the place was infested with pests or disease?

Instinctively we just know places like that are unhealthy. If you wanted to clean up a dank space like that, would your first instinct to be Lysol, Windex, and Ajax? Or would you instead throw open the windows, let in some fresh air and sunlight, and hose the place down?

Our bodies are the same way. Pests and infections tend to thrive in unhealthy environments, but with some fresh air, sunlight, and plenty of clean water to flush us out, our bodies become far less hospitable to disease.

Breathe Deeply

First, let's not even go so far as to talk about fresh air… right now let's just talk about air, period. Americans tend to be a pretty stressed out bunch, and when we get stressed, we often unconsciously quit breathing. Even if this happens only for a few seconds at a time, the effects may be cumulative.

What Happens When You Hold Your Breath

There are a few primary routes for toxin elimination. These include the urinary system, the liver, the bowels, the sweat, and the breath. We breathe in oxygen and breathe out carbon dioxide, in a reciprocal exchange with plants. But when we hold our breath, this delicate balance gets disrupted. Carbon dioxide accumulates in our bodies, which acts as an acid in the bloodstream. A complicated buffer system involving the kidneys has to kick in to buffer this process and keep us from becoming too acidic (the same buffer system that keeps our electrolytes in check). Without this buffering process, we would quickly go into respiratory distress, which can be very serious. Symptoms of respiratory distress include confusion, fatigue, lethargy, shortness of breath, and sleepiness.

(Sound familiar–albeit in milder form?)

What Contributes to Insufficient Breathing?

This can be as simple as the way you are sitting as you stare at your computer (like I am doing right now–I just sat up straighter as I typed this). Proper breathing comes from your belly as your diaphragm lowers, and not from your chest. Hunching over requires you to chest-breathe, which gives you less than adequate respiration.

Another cause, of course, is stress. The autonomic "fight or flight" response leads to short, shallow breathing; "rest and digest" promotes deep belly breathing. Stress can be caused by even something as simple as overwhelming amounts of email (which led to the term, "email apnea". Yes, that's a real thing.) A constant sense of urgency doesn't help you remember to breathe deeply–this is something for which we have to fight.

The Solution

One of the most well-known and least utilized

tricks for coping with anxiety is deep breathing. Sit up straight; put your hand on your belly to remind yourself to breathe from there and not from your chest. Close your eyes, and count as you inhale (and your belly expands) to 8 or 10 or whatever number feels right to you, but don't rush it. Then exhale just as completely, and for the same count. Do this a few times and you will feel yourself become much more relaxed.

It's a good idea to take breaks throughout the day and breathe like this. You may not have to close your eyes and count, as long as you breathe consciously and on purpose. Or, join a gentle stretching or exercise class such as yoga or Tai Chi, where breathing is a central component of the movement. I know I feel a sort of euphoria after these classes, and while some of it is undoubtedly due to the movement itself, much of it is likely due to a greater supply of oxygen to the brain than I typically get!

Drink Water

Sometimes we forget about water as a key component to our health. It's easy to forget, because it's so readily available. But water plays a vital role in almost every system of our bodies. This makes sense, because about 80% of our bodies are comprised of water. Water is about 70% of lean muscle; it makes up about 80% of our blood, and roughly 85% of our brain volume.

The Effect of Water on Blood

When I have a patient with low blood pressure, my first question is, "How much water have you been drinking?" Low fluid intake equals low blood volume. Low blood volume can equal low blood pressure, and thus lower blood flow to your organs (decreasing the supply of oxygen and nutrients and elimination of waste from those tissues). Patients with low blood pressure and blood volume frequently say they experience the room going dark for a few seconds when they stand up too quickly—it takes a bit longer for the blood to get to their brains from the sudden shift in position. (This is also often an indication of adrenal fatigue—see Chapter 13).

The Effect of Water on Toxins

One of the main purposes of water is to assist in the elimination of waste. This happens not just in the bloodstream (because more blood means flushing out those tissues faster), but it also helps to flush out the organs of elimination, such as the liver, kidneys, and bowels. (Think of it this way. When something *not* inside of your body is dirty, what do you use to flush it out?)

Low water intake leads to low urine output and constipation—which means toxins are not getting out of your body effectively. Toxin accumulation can lead to all kinds of symptoms, depending on what the toxin is and where your susceptibilities lie (see Chapters 10-13).

The Symptoms of Dehydration

Low water intake can lead to dehydration, of course, and the symptoms of acute dehydration can be severe and even fatal (including a fast heart rate to compensate for low blood volume and blood pressure, fast breathing to compensate for lower oxygen delivery to the tissues, dry mouth, and eventually loss of consciousness). Symptoms of chronic dehydration include constipation (this is one of the first things to pay attention to if you are constipated—how much water are you drinking?), headache (remember that 85% of our brains are water), and muscle cramping, since dehydration leads to an imbalance in some of the key electrolytes such as magnesium, potassium, chloride, calcium, and sodium. Remember from Chapter 2 that electrolyte imbalances are usually responsible for muscle cramps.

Different Types of Water

All water sources are not created equal. Here's the breakdown of different sources.

Tap Water

We've all heard how contaminated our tap water is. If you're curious to know what's in the water supply near you, go to the Environmental Working Group's website (at http://www.ewg.org/tap-water/whats-in-yourwater.php) and type in your zip code. In my area, the contaminants that exceed health guidelines include arsenic, lead, radioactive alpha particles, and four disinfectant byproducts formed as a result of chlorine or other disinfectants. Quite a few other contaminants were detected below the health limit levels.

So, not the best option. But better than being de-hydrated.

Bottled Water

Although bottled water seems to be cleaner than tap water, according to the NRDC, some 25% of bottled water also contains too-high levels of at least one contaminant.

But more importantly than that, most single-use bottled water is sold in flimsy plastic bottles, a common source of phthalates. Phthalates are not only estrogenic, they have been found to increase programmed cell death (particularly in testicular cells). Overall, phthalates are linked to breast cancer, birth defects, low sperm count, obesity, diabetes, and thyroid problems. (More on this in Chapter 11.)

The stiffer the plastic, however, the less of an issue phthalates become. And 25% is quite a bit better than 100%... so it does seem that delivery-based water services are a better option than tap water.

Leanne had been a patient of mine about a year earlier, and I hadn't seen her in awhile. She returned because suddenly one month, her period became about three times heavier than usual (according to her.) "I'm bleeding like a stuck pig!" she told me.

It seemed very strange that a normal cycle would alter so abruptly in a single month, so I started to ask questions to find out what had changed. Wondering if perhaps she'd had an acute exposure to phthalates, I asked if she'd started using plastics for her food or her water bottle. Her eyes grew wide. "Actually, yes!" She told me the glass water bottle she normally used had broken about a month earlier, and she'd intended to replace it but hadn't gotten around to it. Instead, she'd been using a plastic one she carried in her purse, refilling it daily.

"Bingo," I said. It was June in Tucson, AZ, so the

phthalate content in the water was likely even worse than usual, as the heat encourages pthalates to leech into the water.

I told her to go buy a glass or stainless steel water bottle ASAP, and also prescribed a detox protocol including sauna, hydrotherapy, castor oil packs, and enemas. For good measure, I put her on Chaste Tree to help normalize her cycle.

Sure enough, Leanne's next period returned to normal.

Filtered Water

You can buy pitchers, bottles, or faucet attachments to filter your tap water. These will remove chlorine (and therefore chlorine byproducts), and positively charged ions such as copper, cadmium, mercury, and lead.

Seems to me this is an easy and cheap solution.

Reverse Osmosis Water

Reverse Osmosis water is the best way to ensure that the highest percentage of all contaminants are removed from your water.

The main concern I have with reverse osmosis water is that it also removes necessary minerals like electrolytes, which we most definitely need. That's not concerning to me unless this is all you drink.

Then you might end up with some imbalances. Those who drink mostly reverse osmosis would certainly need an electrolyte replacement of some kind.

Kangen Water

This very expensive filtration system ionizes water, rendering your drinking water alkaline to the tune of 8.5-9.5 pH. The idea is that it will help your body to become more alkaline.

Quick chemistry interlude to address this idea: An acid is any chemical substance that releases a proton ion (H^+). A base is any chemical substance that accepts a proton ion.

Adding more protons to your bloodstream will decrease its pH, so your body has a fancy buffering system to balance them out. The system involves bicarbonate (HCO^{3-}), which is stored in your bones and bound to either calcium or sodium (Ca^+ and Na $^+$), and phosphate (PO_4^-), which is also stored in your bones, complexed with calcium.

When your bloodstream has excess protons (acid), your body pulls some of these basic ions, such as bicarbonate and phosphate, from your bones in order to maintain a pH of 7.35-7.40. But this means your bones lose calcium, because phosphate and bicarbonate are bound to calcium. This is why overtaxing the buffering system can lead to osteoporosis.

Ultimately your kidneys are responsible for getting rid of excess protons and reabsorbing bicarbonate to restore the balance in the blood. In order to do this, they must spill many other ions into the urine, including calcium, and decrease elimination of the negative ion citrate, which helps dissolve calcium. Most kidney stones (75-85%) are made of either calcium oxalate or calcium phosphate. What this means is, there's a direct correlation between the acidic Standard American Diet and the formation of the most common kind of kidney stones.

However, because water has a pH right around 7 (like most of the fluids in your body), it should not activate the buffering systems at all and therefore should not cause a problem. So as far as I can tell, Kangen water systems are unnecessary.

Sunlight

We all pretty much know we feel better outside—there's just something refreshing about being out in nature. Turns out there are good reasons for this.

Vitamin D (some of which is ingested in the diet, but 90-95% of which comes from sunlight) has been the darling of the nutritional world for years now. Here's why.

The Benefits of Vitamin D

- **It's Anti-Cancer.** Over 2000 studies link deficiency of Vitamin D to cancer, and one study[1] suggests that keeping Vitamin D levels at just 40 ng/mL lowers overall cancer risk by about 77%. Another study[2] suggests that a serum level of 55–60 ng/mL may reduce the breast cancer rate by *half* in temperate climates.
- **It lowers the risk of diabetes.** Turns out, vitamin D status is linked more closely to diabetes than is obesity.[3]
- **It lowers the risk of Multiple Sclerosis (MS).** MS occurs a lot less often in sunny places than in dark and gloomy ones.[4]
- **It reduces PMS and period cramping.** Apparently Vitamin D is anti-inflammatory, too.[5] And actually, this suggests any inflammatory condition can improve with a healthy dose of Vitamin D.

Quick Interlude: Why the Chronic Vitamin D Deficiency?

Just about every patient I test is low in Vitamin D unless they're supplementing with it (which by my standards means less than 40 ng/mL—the lab says less than 30 ng/mL is considered deficient). This is the case across the board, even though I live in Arizona where it's sunny nearly all the time, and even with patients who tell me they spend a lot of time in the sun without or with minimal sunscreen. So what gives?

Physiology 101 on Vitamin D

When we're exposed to UVB rays from the sun, our skin creates 7-dehydrocholesterol. This enters the bloodstream and stops off at the liver, where it turns into 25-hydroxyvitamin D. (Alternatively you can eat 25-hydroxyvitamin D from fish, meat, eggs, and cheese.) This is the value tested on labs.

Then this version travels to the kidneys and turns into the more metabolically active form called calcitriol, aka 1,25 dihydroxyvitamin D. Calcitriol's main job is to increase calcium absorption from food.

But here comes the fun part: all of the nutrients in your body are connected to one another, either directly or indirectly. Tamper with one and you can cause repercussions elsewhere. Also, keep in mind that your body is a living system, always seeking balance. So if, for example, your tissue levels of calcium are higher than they should be, your body may shut down calcitriol production in the kidneys to try to achieve that balance.

Why Tissue Burden of Calcium Might be High

Remember that study that came out a few years ago that suggested calcium supplementation could increase the risk of heart attacks?[6] The concern here is that atherosclerotic plaques contain calcium deposits, and perhaps therefore taking calcium in supplement form will contribute to plaque formation. (This refers to non-absorbable forms of calcium taken by themselves, by the way, such as calcium oxide or sulfate, and not to absorbable forms found complexed with other factors for bone deposition or in multivitamins… but the idea that too much calcium can precipitate out onto body tissues is real.[7])

We might have too much calcium in our tissues but not enough in our bones (hence the rampant osteoporosis) due to our highly acidic diets in the US, taxing our blood buffering systems to the max. As mentioned above, the buffering system gets activated in response to substances that have an acidifying effect on the body, in order to maintain the optimum blood pH. Foods with an acidic effect on the body buffering systems include beef, ice cream, canned fruits, peanuts, bacon, tuna, corn, sugar, vinegar, corn syrup, cereals, mustard, mayo, corn tortillas, milk, sardines, soft drinks, artificial sweeteners, and ketchup.

Foods with an alkalinizing effect include alfalfa, celery, barley grass, peppers, beet greens, broccoli, cabbage, mustard greens, chard greens, collard greens, chlorella, onions, cucumber, spinach, spirulina, garlic, green beans, dandelions, lettuce, kohlrabi, kale, pumpkin, wheat grass, sprouts, watercress, and wild greens.

So basically our calcium is in the wrong place: it's in our tissues rather than our bones, because our bodies have pulled it from our bones in order to counteract our highly acidic diets. This may dial down our vitamin D production, even in the presence of adequate sunlight: because our bodies are saying, "Stop with the calcium already!"

Vitamin K and Calcium

Vitamin K is another fat-soluble vitamin like Vitamin D, and its job is to allow the body to take calcium and use it in the clotting cascade. Vitamin K also produces a protein called osteocalcin, which puts calcium into the bones.

You get vitamin K1 from super-healthy veggies (broccoli, turnips, cabbage, cauliflower, and spinach), and then it gets converted to the active Vitamin K2 by the good bacteria in your gut. But alas, most of us aren't eating those veggies, and we also don't have nearly as much good bacteria in our guts as we ought to (and often we have a lot of bad bacteria instead).

Result: too little vitamin K —> too much calcium in the tissues (rather than in the bones and clotting cascade, where it's supposed to be.)

How Magnesium is connected to Calcium and Vitamin D

Like Vitamin D, magnesium also helps to regulate calcium levels, because magnesium and calcium have opposite effects. (Calcium and magnesium should remain in about a 2:1 ratio.) But if you don't have enough magnesium (and it's a common deficiency, as addressed in Chapter 2), your tissue levels of calcium go up, too.

Magnesium is also used in the metabolism of Vitamin D, so too little magnesium can lead to low Vitamin D that way, also.

So, while it is important to get enough sunlight

for adequate Vitamin D production, I hope you're getting the message that *all healthy habits work together in concert.* In order for sunlight's production of Vitamin D to be as effective as possible, you also need to consume a healthy diet and balance your micronutrients.

The sun does more than just boost your Vitamin D levels, though.

Some forms of depression are directly linked to low Vitamin D (Seasonal Affective Disorder) but even aside from that, **sun exposure boosts serotonin,** the "feel-good" neurotransmitter.

One study[6] shows that exposure to UVB rays increases production if nitric oxide, which causes blood vessels to dilate, thus **lowering blood pressure.**

Exposure to sunlight early in the morning helps your body to produce melatonin earlier, making it **easier to sleep** at the end of the day.[7]

The Take-Home Message:

- **Drink clean, filtered water.** Half your body weight in ounces is a good rule of thumb (so if you weigh 140 lbs, you should be drinking 80 oz of water daily), but you should increase that number if you are out in the summer heat or exercising (which you should be—see chapter 6!) This is one of the simplest and most important things you can do for your health.

- **Breathe deeply!** This helps your body to remain alkaline.
- **Eat whole foods,** to minimize acidity in your body. Follow the bullet points at the end of Chapter 1 for this!
- **Spend 5-15 minutes a day in the sun, without sunblock, three times per week in the spring and summertime (and an hour in the winter).** Longer sun exposures aren't necessary—there are diminishing returns after that point, increasing the risk of aging from the sun and skin cancers, but not improving Vitamin D Status. This will help to boost your Vitamin D levels, boost your serotonin, boost your nitric oxide, lower inflammation, and generally make you healthier!

CHAPTER 5

Building Block #5: Sleep

We all feel better when we get enough sleep.

But sometimes it's hard to prioritize sleep when there are other things you'd rather accomplish, or things that have to get done. According to the CDC, some 40% of Americans are chronically sleep deprived[1]—defined as unintentionally nodding off at least once during the previous month!

Getting adequate sleep for your age and body is one of the absolute foundational health requirements. Here are some of the things plenty of sleep does for you (and that lack of sleep can deprive you of):

Sleep improves your memory. Remember those commercials years ago when Candace Bergen that every time you learn something, it makes a new "wrinkle in your brain?" This reorganization of the brain's structure when both learning something new and consolidating that memory is known as *neuroplasticity*, and sleep seems to be a necessary part of this process. You may even practice new skills in your dreams, which strengthens that new neural pathway and makes those same skills easier to perform in your waking hours.

On the other hand, why does sleep deprivation cause memory problems? One possible (chilling) explanation is that sleep gives your brain time to "clean up" toxic proteins that can accumulate throughout waking hours, including beta amyloid and tau—the proteins linked with Alzheimer's Disease. In one study[2], mice who were only allowed to sleep four hours per night were not only impaired in their ability to recall and learn new tasks, they were found to have an increased level of tau in their brains.

Sleep helps you live longer. The reasons for this are not entirely clear, but it may have to do with the hormone melatonin (the "sleep hormone"), which is a powerful antioxidant, among other things. Insufficient sleep is also correlated with higher levels of inflammation, and therefore higher incidence of hypertension and cardiovascular disease. Even in the short term, sleep deprivation is correlated with dramatically reduced immune function.

Sleep helps you lose weight. Consistently getting less than 6 hours of sleep per night is correlated with a higher BMI (basal metabolic index)—which means it's harder to lose weight if you're not sleeping enough. This is because during sleep, your body secretes hormones that regulate appetite and blood sugar. Insufficient sleep leads to an increase in the hormone ghrelin (think of your stomach growling—this is a hunger hormone), a decrease in leptin (the opposite of ghrelin), and an increase in cortisol, the stress hormone, which (among other things) increases your blood sugar. Lack of sleep can therefore lead to obesity, poor blood sugar control, and even diabetes. (Conversely, 8 hours of sleep per night is correlated with a lower BMI.)

Sleep improves performance, at whatever you do—be it athletics, school, work, or creative endeavors. This probably has to do with that feeling of drowsiness, which is at least partly due to the accumulation of adenosine, a by-product of neuronal activity which builds up during waking hours and leads to the feeling of being tired. (By the way, caffeine works by blocking the adenosine receptors, as well as indirectly pumping out more adrenaline to keep you going even when your adenosine levels are high.)

Sleep prevents accidents. Probably also in part due to the accumulation of adenosine in the brain, driving under the effects of drowsiness is responsible for 20 percent of all car accidents, causing 8000 deaths yearly in the US. In some cases it is considered even more dangerous than driving under the influence of alcohol.

Sleep helps to restore and rejuvenate tissues. Many physiologic activities are reduced during sleep, but some are increased. One such activity is the release of growth hormone (GH), which helps to repair muscles and tissues from the normal wear-and-tear of everyday living. (For this reason, conditions like fibromyalgia, or chronic muscle pain, are correlated with insufficient sleep—and therefore insufficient GH to repair muscles.)

Adequate Sleep

How much sleep do you need to reap these benefits and avoid these pitfalls? According to the National Sleep Foundation, there's a range based on your age and your genetics.

- *Newborns (0-3 mo):* 14-17 hours is average, but the range can go anywhere from 11-19 hours
- *Infants (4-11 mo):* 12-15 hours average, 10-18 hours may apply
- *Toddlers (1-2 years):* 11-14 hours average, 9-16 hours may apply
- *Preschool (3-5 years):* 10-13 hours average, 8-14 hours may apply
- *School age (6-13 years):* 9-11 hours average, 7-12 hours may apply
- *Teenagers (14-17 years):* 8-10 hours average, 7-11 hours may apply
- *Young adults (18-25 years):* 7-9 hours average, 6-11 hours may apply
- *Adults (26-64 years):* 7-9 hours average, 6-10 hours may apply
- *Older adults (65 and over):* 7-8 hours average, 5-9 hours may apply.

My advice on finding the right number of hours for you: on a day when you're not already sleep-deprived (i.e. suffering from some of the side effects above), turn off your alarm and see how many hours you sleep. That's probably your ideal number. Our world doesn't really make it easy to sleep nine hours per night as an adult, so I recommend finding an average number at which you can function well and sticking to it. For example: if nine is ideal for you, but you can function well on eight and any less than that will put you in a deficit over time, then make eight your minimum. Every now and then things come up and you won't even be able to achieve eight, though. If that happens, do a little math for the subsequent nights that week. If one night you only get five hours, then you're at a deficit of three—so you need to get those three in over the rest of the week, plus your eight for each of the subsequent nights. That means you can either sleep eleven the very next night, or ten the next night and nine the night after, or nine the three following nights.

That should be enough to help you average out, and prevent the deficits from stacking up.

Good Sleep Hygiene

If you struggle with insomnia, before trying all the fancy supplements and medications out there to help you nod off, make sure you've done all the basic stuff first.

Try to go to bed at the same time every night and wake up at the same time every morning, even if you're not tired at night and/or got very little sleep by morning. It is best to wake with the sun in order to reset your biological clock, spend a few minutes in the early morning sunlight, and then go to bed early enough that this will give you as many hours as you need to feel your best. Night shift workers need to maintain as regular a schedule as possible to give their internal clocks a chance to adjust, and many of them may adjust faster if they sleep before going to work instead of after, or nap beforehand as well as after, in order to mimic the normal shift schedule of going to work shortly after rising.

If you cannot fall asleep, get up and do something else. The anxiety of trying to fall asleep can actually exacerbate the problem.

The last hour (or at least half an hour) before you go to bed, do something very calming— read a book, listen to music, pray, or meditate in bed until you start to nod off. Try not to watch TV or stare at a computer screen right before bed. Do not take any stimulants or engage in stimulating activities before bed.

Have a cup of tea (chamomile is my favorite) while you do this, and try to slow down your breathing. Alternatively, you can try having a cup of warm (organic!) milk right before bed, with a pinch of nutmeg or turmeric. If you are sensitive to dairy, try warm soy milk (non-GMO!), almond milk, flax milk, rice milk, or hemp milk instead.

Consume little or no alcohol before bedtime. Alcohol may help you fall into a light sleep, but it maintains only lighter stages and prevents REM and deeper stages of sleep. This means you can be awakened more easily. This is why drinking alcohol before bed is associated with waking in the middle of the night.

Give up smoking. Like those who have night caps right before bed, smokers tend to sleep very lightly, and wake after 3-4 hours of sleep due to the nicotine withdrawal.

Avoid caffeine after 2 pm. Although the half life of caffeine in the bloodstream is four hours in theory, this depends on the individual's metabolic rate. Some people process caffeine faster and some slower. It's best to err on the side of caution.

Are you taking supplements right before bed? Make sure there are no stimulants in them. This includes B vitamins and even vitamin C for some patients.

Get enough exercise: 20-30 minutes per day.

Keep your room cool—you lose your ability to regulate body temperature during REM, so abnormally hot or cold temperatures in the environment can disrupt this stage of sleep.

Some people have difficulty sleeping due to an overabundance of thoughts. If you find that you cannot help but continue to problem-solve, **get out of bed and write your thoughts down on a piece of paper** until you can think of no more.

Resist getting up to go to the bathroom if you wake up in the middle of the night. Bladders are always full at night, but it shouldn't wake you up, nor should it keep you awake. Usually when you feel like you have to go, if you ignore it, you will drift off to sleep anyway.

Put the bedroom clock out of arm's reach and facing away from you so you can't see it. This may help for two reasons: one, it decreases the anxiety associated with the hour, and two, some people are especially light sensitive and need total darkness to sleep their best. The light can actually disrupt the production of melatonin.

Have a light snack before bedtime so you're not hungry. Hunger is a cause of insomnia in many animals, including humans.

Try not to nap much after 2 pm if possible.

The Right Kind of Sleep

Although we hear about REM sleep more often than other stages because it is associated with dreams, there are actually five stages of sleep: 1, 2, 3, 4, and REM, which occurs between stages 1 and 2. Stages 3 and 4 are the deepest stages. Without adequate sleep in stages 3 and 4, people wake feeling groggy and "hung over"—even if you hit your ideal number of hours. My favorite natural remedy to get people into stages 3 and 4 (assuming they're already not drinking alcohol before bedtime—if so, cut that out) is the amino acid and neurotransmitter glycine[3]. I usually recommend a powdered version, since it's easier to take a lot of it; 3 grams an hour before bedtime works well to help propel patients into REM and stage 3-4 sleep.

More stubborn cases of insomnia may require individual neurotransmitter testing and supplementation based on lab results, hormone balancing, and/or individualized homeopathic prescriptions. For patients who have never been on long-term sleep medications, this is usually sufficient. For patients who already have a dependency on sleep meds such as Ambien, Lorazepam, Trazodone, Lunesta, etc—it's possible to get off, but it's usually a process of finding the right taper schedule combined with the right additional supplements to help reset your body's natural sleep cycle. Long-term sleep medication users typically require a long drawn out taper process, so be patient.

CHAPTER 6

Building Block #6: Exercise

It can be hard to start a new routine. But if you can find a buddy to help keep you accountable and motivated for those first 21 days (which is about the length of time necessary to create a new habit), regular exercise is probably the very best thing you can do to improve your mood, and one of the biggest changes you can make to improve your joint health, lose weight, lower blood pressure and cholesterol levels, and of course, look and feel better! Here's a quick run-down of why exercise can improve each of those things.

Exercise and Your Mood

The endorphins released with vigorous exercise are very similar chemically to morphine, which can decrease sensitivity to pain and even induce euphoria —hence the idea of the "runner's high". Exercise also promotes better blood flow throughout the body, including the brain—improving your overall sense of well-being, and bringing the necessary precursors the brain needs to build mood-enhancing neurotransmitters.

Exercise and Your Joints

Your blood is your body's nutrient delivery system. Because of that, most parts of your body are supplied with blood directly by their own blood vessels and system of capillaries, bringing nutrients and oxygen and eliminating waste. If the blood supply is cut off for any reason, the tissue on the other end starts to die.

Your cartilage in your joints is an exception to this: it doesn't have its own direct blood supply. This is partly why it doesn't heal as quickly after injury as other tissues do. Instead, it gets its nutrients by diffusion. This requires movement. Too little blood, and eventually the cartilage starves and dies.

Continuous movement of between five and twenty minutes at a time stimulates the chondrocytes (cells that produce cartilage) to generate more of it. This is why exercise is just about the best thing you can do to prevent the joint pain that comes from loss of cartilage. Exercise will also help you lose weight, of course—which means less strain on weight-bearing joints.

Exercise and Your Digestion

Bowel irregularity is unfortunately super common in industrialized countries. Much of this has to do with the SAD (Standard American Diet), which is high in processed foods and sugar, and low in fiber. However, the more exercise you get, the more toned your core muscles become and the better your bowels tend to move.

If you hate exercise, it's probably just because you're not used to it. Everyone can find some form of physical activity that they enjoy if they're determined. Do you love the beauty of nature? Go for a walk in the evening when it gets cool, or in the morning as the sun rises. Do you enjoy calming stretches? Sign up for a yoga class. Do you enjoy fluid movement? Consider taking up dancing! How about slow hikes? Really, there's something for everyone. Start slow, but make it a habit. That's the key.

Okay, on to the specifics. The three components of fitness are aerobic (cardiovascular), strength, and flexibility. Most forms of physical activity will provide some benefits in all three areas.

Aerobic

Aerobic exercises are those that involve repetitive motions of large muscle groups. These include walking, jogging, swimming, bicycling, Elliptical machines, aerobics classes, dancing, hiking, and rowing machines. Here's how to do it right.

Before you start, calculate your target heart rate zone to make sure you achieve the benefits of aerobic exercise. Maximum heart rate can be calculated as approximately 220 beats per minute, minus your age. Multiply this number by 0.6 in order to yield 60% of your maximum heart rate, or by 0.8 in order to yield 80% of your maximum heart rate. **The target heart rate range for maximum benefits is 60-80%.** As long as you keep your heart beating at a rate of between 60-80% for at least 20 minutes, the benefits of aerobic exercise will be attained.

The easiest way to determine your heart rate is to count the number of beats in 15 seconds (measured at the wrist or in the neck) and multiply by four to give beats per minute. For example, if you count 22 beats in 15 seconds, your heart rate would be 88 (22 x 4) bpm. You can perform this calculation while exercising to determine whether you are in the desired range, or you can use exercise monitors specifically designed to measure this for you.

The intensity of exercise required to reach your target heart rate will vary according to your level of fitness when you begin your exercise program. If you have not exercised in some time, it won't take a lot of work to reach your target heart rate.

Any intense exercise should incorporate a warm up and cool down period. A warm up can be simply beginning your exercise at low intensity and gradually increasing to your desired intensity over five minutes. This prepares your body for aerobic exercise and prevents injuries.

Strength

Begin a strength training program that works all of the major muscle groups of the upper and lower body. Below is a list of exercises that fall into these categories. Ask the trainers at your gym to identify these machines for you if you are unfamiliar with them.

Upper body exercises include bicep curls, tricep

extensions, lat pull downs, seated rows, chest press/ fly, shoulder press, and upright rows.

Lower body exercises include the leg press, squats, or lunges; leg curls, calf raises, and abdominal crunches.

A repetition is the number of times you repeat a particular exercise. Each time you complete this number of repetitions, it's called a set. If your goal is to lose weight or create lean muscle, lower weight and higher repetitions is recommended, while higher weight and fewer repetitions are preferred to bulk up. As a rule of thumb, most trainers recommend three sets of each exercise, with 8 to 12 repetitions.

Repetitions should be slow—lift to a count of 2 and hold at the top of the contraction for about 1 second. Lower to the count of 4. Going faster while lifting or lowering the resistance uses momentum, not muscle, which both increases the chance of injury and decreases effectiveness of the exercise.

Rest your muscles in between sets. 60-90 seconds is recommended for muscle recovery. Alternatively, in order to save time, I use my "rest" period to perform another exercise using a different muscle group (called a superset). Usually I choose the muscle group that does the opposite of the one I just worked (or the antagonistic muscle group)—for instance, I will superset bicep curls with tricep extensions.

Work each muscle group until you can't lift the weight any more without a rest. Trainers call this working the muscle to fatigue. This will ensure that you get the maximum benefits from your exercise.

Perform strength training on a given muscle group only every other day. It takes two days for your muscles to heal from microtears incurred during strength training. Many trainers recommend strength training only three days per week. Alternatively, I do some strength training daily but alternate between back/chest, upper and lower body workouts.

Increase your resistance as you gain strength. If you stop increasing resistance, your gains will plateau. This is fine, however, if you've achieved your desired level of fitness.

Stretching

Most of us think of stretching as something you

do for maybe 15 seconds before you work out, to prevent muscle injury. But there's a lot more to it than that.

So many of my patients complain of neck and back pain, which nearly always starts with tight muscles. Muscles can become tight due to posture problems, overuse, repetitive movements that strain one part of the body and cause compensation elsewhere, and (often) stress—which causes us to hunch up or hunch over, as our bodies unconsciously bear our burdens for us.

Much of this could be prevented with regular stretching!

Stretching will increase blood flow. Some cultures think of blood as the "life force" of a creature, and for good reason: blood brings oxygen and nutrients to cells, and eliminates metabolic waste. So many great naturopathic therapies (also including hydrotherapy and massage) boil down to this: increased circulation = increased vitality. This goes for all forms of exercise too, by the way.

Stretching leads to greater flexibility. Think of it this way: if you drop a glass bottle on the ground, it shatters, because (among other things) glass has no "give". It can't absorb the impact. Conversely, if you drop a rubber ball on the ground, it bounces, because rubber can absorb the impact. You want your muscles to be more like rubber than like glass. Flexibility = "give."

Stretching increases your range of motion. The more range of motion you have, the better your balance becomes. Better balance will not only make you more graceful, but it will also prevent injury from falls.

Stretching leads to greater strength gains. Stretching may actually improve muscular performance and endurance, much the way lifting weights does.

Stretching is great for stress reduction. It forces you to slow down and breathe deeply, for one thing. It also decreases some of the secondary signs of stress, such as shoulder and neck tightness. But, as a side benefit to increased blood flow, stretching also releases the same endorphins you get from other forms of exercise—which is why a yoga class can leave you feeling euphoric!

Tips for Stretching Right

Make sure you warm up first. Contrary to popular opinion, stretching itself is not a warm-up. A "warm up" is an activity that increases blood flow to the muscles. Stretching a muscle that doesn't yet have that extra influx of oxygen from increased blood flow can actually cause injury. It's a better idea to stretch your muscles after your workout, instead of before... or to at least "warm up" with some light cardio before stretching.

Stretch for symmetry. Especially if one side of your body tends to have issues more than the other (which is most of us,) stretching can help to minimize stiffness, maximize range of motion, and prevent further compensatory problems down the line.

Hold the stretch for 30-60 seconds. You want to give plenty of time for the muscle to respond appropriately. Tighter muscles will need a longer stretch.

The Take-Home Message:

- Incorporate some form of aerobic exercise, strength training, and stretching every week.
- Shoot for a minimum of 30 minutes of aerobic exercise at your fitness level, three times per week.

- Shoot for a minimum of two strength training sessions per week at 15 minutes each.
- Either do some stretching after every workout, or make it a practice to attend a yoga, pilates, or Tai chi class once or twice a week.

CHAPTER 7

Building Block #7: Recreation

One man's recreation is another man's work.

Personally I can't stand Sudoku (probably because I am not very good with numbers). Not a big fan of crossword puzzles, either. But I know several people who think both are very relaxing. I have patients who despise all forms of exercise, yet I have others who participate in bodybuilding competitions for the sheer pleasure of it. Some of my friends think of cooking as a chore, and others are gourmet chefs, regularly hosting dinner parties in their spare time.

But here's the question. What do you spend most of your time doing? Does it recharge you, or deplete you? And if it depletes you, what (if anything) are you doing to refuel?

Many people now struggle with ADT, or Attention Deficit Trait—a product of our fast-paced environment. Due to high-pressure, noisy work environments requiring multitasking in order to get anything done, these people increasingly find it difficult to prioritize, stay organized, and manage their time effectively. Some of the problems associated with ADT are decreased productivity, insomnia, anxiety, irritability, and fatigue—particularly adrenal fatigue (which comes from long term stress; see Chapter 16).

Activity that habitually "depletes" you is stressful almost by definition. One of the most important mediators for stress due to overwork is to take at least 24 consecutive hours off from what you consider "work" every week, and choose instead to do what you consider "fun."

Taking a "Sabbath" Rest

This concept is not new. One of, if not the earliest, mentions of it showed up in Judaic law (what is now the Old Testament in Christianity), requiring the Jews to take 24 hours off of work every Saturday, from sun up to sun down. Prior to this time, the Jews had been enslaved by the Egyptians for 400 years, during which time they worked 7 days a week, 365 days a year. Originally the Sabbath was meant to be a gift to them, enabling them to rest without feeling guilty for "slacking off."

But by the time Jesus showed up, the religious leaders had attached many additional rules to what did and did not constitute "work," making the Sabbath into a chore, rather than a true day of rest. Jesus (angrily) told them they were totally missing the spirit of the command—God intended to save them from the overwork from which He had originally delivered them.

The point is, rest looks different for everyone. But the ultimate goal is to recharge from life's depleting effects, so that we can return to our regular world and act more effectively than before.

Obviously, sleep is one of the best ways to recharge. Getting enough sleep is fundamental, but it's amazing how often we manage to convince ourselves that we don't really need it that much. Hopefully Chapter 5 convinced you otherwise. We need a good night's sleep—every night.

You can also replenish yourself by enjoying what you've worked for! One of my new favorite handouts to give patients was inspired by Stephen Covey's "7 Habits of Highly Effective People," and it is the "urgent vs important" chart.[1] It's a tool to help differentiate between those activities that are truly important (meaning the consequences of not doing them will be severe) versus those activities that are merely urgent (meaning people are yelling at us to do them ASAP —or we are yelling at ourselves—but it really won't matter that much in the long run if we let them slide.) Activities that fall under the "not urgent but important" category are those that allow us to develop the life we truly desire to lead. They are things like enjoying family and friends, engaging in hobbies we love, getting healthy, and serving others. These are the activities that refuel us, rather than deplete us.

Have some unstructured time. This is time to do whatever you feel like doing, and it will be different for each person. It's most restorative to take a 24 consecutive hours off every week; without it, you can predispose yourself to illness the following week (because chronic stress depletes the immune system). I give this "prescription" to my Type A patients who approach life from the perspective that "there's always more to do!" They are right, there is always more that could be done—and this is the very reason why it's so important to prioritize time off. Work will always expand to fill the time you give it.

Finding a hobby can be critical if you dislike your job, or find it draining. What do you love to do? What would you have done if other "practical" concerns hadn't gotten in the way? This doesn't necessarily have to be a side project, though it can be. If you are an extreme extrovert and you have a desk job that allows for little social interaction, this might look like intentionally cultivating more interpersonal time. If you are an introvert and you are in sales or something that requires lots of face time with others (or if you're a parent and you're with the kids all day long), this might mean intentionally setting aside time to be alone.

During your alone time, maybe consider reading or watching something humorous. Smiling and laughing is a great way to recharge. There is always the "chicken or the egg" question when it comes to mood—are you sad because your "happy" neuro-transmitters are low, or are your neurotransmitters low because you are sad? Either way, the evidence shows that your facial expression not only reflects your mood, but also influences it.[2] Smiling and laughing make you feel happier, even if at first you only do it out of sheer willpower. (Caveat here, though: this does not mean you should suppress your negative emotions, as suppression can be dangerous. It just means you should not wallow in them. More on this in Chapter 9.)

There are Seasons for Everything

I realize it isn't always possible to take a full 24

hours off, or to take evenings off all the time. If you're building a new business, you will probably have to put in a lot of extra hours. If you're in graduate school, you probably won't have much of a social life (or if you do, you probably won't do too well in school!) If you've got a toddler at home with special needs, it might be a few years before you can really take much time for yourself.

The key is recognizing within yourself whether your season of intense work with little downtime has turned into a lifestyle. This can easily occur, especially if that period of intense work has gone on long enough to turn into a habit. We've conditioned ourselves to think, "If I don't put in those extra hours, someone else at the office will get the promotion!", or "If I just work a little longer, I'll get X many new clients, which will translate into more money, more security, or more prestige" …or even, "If I don't continue to put in overtime, I might lose my job, and then who will feed my family?"

It takes wisdom to navigate these situations. You probably know within yourself whether you have turned a season of overwork into a lifestyle of overwork. If you don't know, consider asking someone you trust (and who does not have a vested interest in the answer) whether they believe you have done this and if it's time to begin setting some boundaries.

* * *

Vacation is Productive!

If you are chronically overworked, you will almost certainly notice an increase in your productivity when you listen to the cry of your body and your mind for rest, recreation, and fun. Often, mild cases of insomnia and anxiety, digestive disturbances, tension headaches, irritability and the like will spontaneously resolve with a little R&R. If this is you, take it as your body's cue that you're overdoing it. Time to cut back.

According to the LA Times, over 50% of Americans go more than a year without a vacation (defined as a week off of work, and more than 100 miles from home).[3] This is the lowest percentage in four decades. Surveys have found that this is because workers fear they'll be considered expendable if they take time off, they're gunning for a promotion, they fear the avalanche of work upon their return, or they think no one else can do their job while they're gone.

According to Time Magazine, of those who do go on vacation, 61% of us still do some work while we're there![4] In this day and age of constant connectivity, it's hard to completely unplug. But working really long hours and skipping vacations can have disastrous health effects.

The famous Framingham Study shows that home-makers who take a vacation from being stay-at-home moms every 6 years or less (because let's face it, most of them take their kids with them wherever they go) have twice the risk of heart attacks compared to those who vacation twice per year or more.[5] Also, regular work days of 10 + hours increase the risk of heart attack by 80% in both sexes.[6]

Unless you really love your job, long grueling days tend to sap your joy and make you more prone to anxiety and meltdowns. Compared to those who worked a normal 7-8 hour day, those who regularly work 11 hour shifts have twice the risk of major de-pression.[7]

Henrietta came to me with severe back pain managed with opiates, and fatigue so crushing that she sometimes had to pull over when she drove, for fear that she might wreck. We spent most of the first visit talking about her job: she was a music teacher in a dangerous part of town, under an excessively harsh administration. She worked very long hours, took her work home with her, and felt powerless as her bosses continually demanded more. "But there isn't much demand for music teachers," she told me. "What else can I do? Where else can I go?"

For several visits we simply chased symptoms, with small gains. Finally I told Henrietta a personal story from my own family: years ago, my dad's job was thankless and demanded long hours. They called him in the middle of the night. His bosses took credit for things he'd done.

Unexpectedly he was diagnosed with pancreatic cancer. Two weeks later, he was gone.

I warned Henrietta not to let her job take more from her than she was willing to give.

For whatever reason, that story hit home. Henrietta applied for other jobs, and within a few months, she found one. She had to move to take it, but she's never been happier. The fatigue completely resolved, and the last time I talked to her, she told me she had no back pain as long as she stuck to her exercise routine. For the first time in as long as she could remember, Henrietta said she was doing things she enjoyed, and she looks forward to getting up in the morning.

If declining mental health wasn't bad enough, working too much makes you dumber. The Whitehall II Study study shows that reasoning and creativity drops as work weeks climb above 55 hours.[8] Makes sense, right? Long hours make it harder to think straight.

The message here, obviously, is to take a vacation. But in order to maximize its restorative capacity, choose one that isn't just lounging on the beach. Vacations involving learning new skills are especially good for recharging your batteries.[9]

So go learn a new skill! Take cooking classes. Go on a yoga retreat. Learn to surf or ski. Pick up a new language. Learn to paint. Have an adventure you can take home with you!

And Now, For Some Perspective

Your recreational time is bound to include social functions or family get-togethers: moments you want to enjoy but may be spending with people who do not share your lifestyle. Different diets and lifestyles are normal and need not create stress in what would otherwise be a fun, relaxing situation. Here, too, the key is balance.

When I was a naturopathic medical student, surrounded by other naturopathic students making the same healthy choices that I was, I didn't realize how different my lifestyle had become from the societal "norm".

Once I graduated and rejoined the rest of the population socially, though, I realized that I couldn't be dogmatic anymore—particularly about my food choices, because so many social activities involve food. If I insisted on eating only unprocessed whole foods free of trans fats, chemicals, and added sugar, the people around me would feel judged, even if I didn't consciously intend it. But on the other hand, I didn't want to compromise my health, and I knew too much to think it truly wouldn't make a difference in the long run.

It helps to try and think about it from the other person's perspective, though. Younger people who haven't lived long enough to accumulate much damage yet tend to give almost no thought to nutrition (unless they happen to have a slower metabolism and are concerned about weight gain, or have symptoms so immediate and so severe that they cannot ignore them). I have a patient who knows certain common food additives, like MSG and carrageenan, trigger her migraines, so she has to be meticulous about reading labels, and avoiding most processed foods. But anyone with a less severe reaction would be considered ridiculous for such attention, would they not? Why go to such effort for no apparent gain?

Even some older adults disregard nutrition as long as symptoms are relatively mild and decently controlled with medications. It might not seem like a big deal to have that soda with a meal, or even to choose the salad dressing that has sugar listed as its second ingredient. Of course, it adds up—on average, every American consumes nearly *156 pounds of added sugar per year.*[10] But in the moment, what's one more dessert? For most people, it isn't until their symptoms have become very severe indeed that they're willing to consider the impact of their lifestyle choices on their health. Until then, the benefits of change just don't appear to be worth the sacrifice. This is very human: most of us will resist change until the moment when the pain of changing becomes lower than the pain of staying the same. (I'll bet you can identify at least one negative area in your own life where you're resisting change for exactly this reason.)

But on the flip side, our bodies are amazingly resilient for the most part. If you're generally conscious about your health, and you're blessed with a constitution that is not as sensitive as my patient mentioned above, then one soda, one sugary condiment or one extra dessert won't have a severe impact. Like anything else, it's a cost/benefit analysis. Is sticking to your diet or your principles worth offending your dinner host? Unless you have a serious restriction (i.e. you have Celiac disease and they're serving pizza), in my opinion the answer is generally no. I don't feel great after I eat junk food either, so I try not to do it if I can help it. But sometimes the social capital is more important—provided I'm not in a position to make that compromise too regularly.

The Take-Home Message:

- **Take vacations.** At least once a year, for heaven's sake.

- **Schedule at least 24 hours off every week.** That means you're only allowed to do things you enjoy during that time, only things that recharge you. They don't have to be a consecutive 24 hours, although if you can manage that I would highly recommend it. Consecutive time off is much more restorative than a little here, a little there.
- **Make time for things you love!** These should actually get scheduled into your week, if you're a workaholic. That way you'll actually do them.
- **Try not to be too rigid,** for you perfectionists out there. It's good to eat healthy most of the time, of course! But if you're invited to a party and you know they'll be serving Papa John's, unless you have major health reasons why you shouldn't, go and have a slice. (If you want to, not just to please other people!) Or if you do have major health reasons why you shouldn't, then eat something at home first, and still go! :)

CHAPTER 8

Building Block #8: Solid Relationships

Healthy relationships can be defined by two general rules:

1. We must be able to share with another person (or group of people) who we really are, flaws and all.

2. The other person (or group) must be willing to love and accept us as we are, without criticism or judgment.

If we've internalized enough acceptance and connection over time, we can handle rejection or loss and still continue to offer our true selves in other relationships in the future. But if we haven't, eventually we shut down. Shutting down precludes all possibility of healing relationships—because of course, we have to be willing to show others who we are before they can decide whether or not to love us.

There are many disabling behaviors that indicate a pattern of shutting down; these are the ones I encounter most frequently in my practice. See if you recognize yourself in any of them.

Addictions happen when we use a surrogate to try and fill a real need—and we can use almost anything (including substances, shopping, gambling, sex, and food). You might have an addiction if you seek a surrogate like one of these to relieve negative emotions, especially if you never feel like you've had enough of it. Another red flag might be if one of these surrogates consumes a lot of your resources (mentally, emotionally, financially, or physically). Jesus said in Luke 12:34, "For where your treasure is, there will your heart be also."

Ever found yourself craving sugar and white carbs around mid-afternoon or the evening, especially when you're depressed or feeling down? If so, you are likely self-medicating: these foods help our bodies to produce the neurotransmitter serotonin.

Self-sufficiency says, "I don't need you anyway." It might start out looking like sour grapes, but over time it moves into true denial of the need for other people. Denial tends to keep us "stuck" and therefore isolated, because obviously if we don't realize we need others, we're not about to open up to them (which means it's impossible for us to receive what we really need from them—their love).

Perfectionism. The logic tends to be, "If I were only more (fill in the blank), then they would love me." The trouble is, perfectionists can never relax. Every compliment sounds to their ears like an expectation to do even better the next time. There is usually a lot of fear surrounding the idea that at some point, others will find out who they really are, and they will lose love as a result.

People-pleasing. People pleasers tend to be chameleons; who they are, what they like, and what they will or won't tolerate depends on whom they happen to be with at the time. They often have a hard time saying no, fearing that setting limits will provoke anger and thus, lose love.

If you've adopted protective mechanisms, you've adopted them for a reason. They're symptoms, telling you that there's a problem hiding underneath that still needs to be healed. One of the primary tenets of naturopathic medicine is to *treat the root cause, rather than the symptom.* If you try to discipline yourself to kick your addiction, or to stop wanting admiration, or to stop putting so much pressure on yourself, you'll only be frustrated. If the underlying reason for those protective mechanisms hasn't been addressed, willpower simply won't work. The instinct for self-preservation is too strong.

What does work, in a word, is grace. Only the first of the two conditions for healthy relationships depends upon us (sharing who we really are), but we must do our part. We have to risk showing our less-than-perfect sides to safe people. It's important to choose someone with whom to share who is not likely to be overly critical—support groups or churches are a great place to start. When you've internalized enough love and acceptance from safe relationships, life's inevitable losses and rejections will be much easier to take and you will be more comfortable seeking relationships in the future.

Some people, on the other hand, are relationship seekers by nature. If they have not established the habits and attitudes that are necessary for healthy, functional relationships, they soon end up feeling misunderstood, unappreciated, and, often, trapped. This feeling of powerlessness in a relationship arises from an inability to find the balance we seek. Specifically, we feel powerless when we don't think we can say no without suffering some consequence (damaging a relationship, losing a job, feeling guilty, etc), we desperately desire a particular outcome that we believe is outside our control, or we don't see any way out of a negative or toxic environment, either at work or home or elsewhere.

Setting Boundaries

The biggest power issue I tend to see in my practice (and one I've struggled with myself!) is guilt. "Isn't it selfish to say no when I could say yes?" we ask.

On one hand, helping others is one of the most fulfilling experiences in life. It is good to look out for the interests of others, and not just for our own. If we have the resources to help, and we want to help, then we should help.

But that "want to" is key—the whole thing hinges on the concept of choice. **In order to say yes from your heart, you first have to have the ability to say no.** If you don't feel like "no" is an option, then a "yes" can only come from compulsion (not from love). If you find yourself frequently saying yes when you want to say no, you are not actually being selfless—you're being hypocritical.

The Apostle Paul says that we should each give "what [we have] decided in [our hearts] to give, not reluctantly or under compulsion, for God loves a cheerful giver" (2 Corinthians 9:7). Saying yes when you really mean no breeds resentment, and can cause you to withdraw from a person who makes demands (the "passive aggressive" approach), which damages relationships far more than simply saying what you mean. Over time this sort of disconnect between who you really are and who you present yourself to be can also lead to problems with anxiety. (Remember, emotions are symptoms of a problem, and not the problem itself!)

A prerequisite for any healthy relationship is freedom. So let your "yes be yes, and your no be no" (Matthew 5:37).

It is important to keep in mind, however, that even if you are agreeing to something that comes easily from your heart, there is always the possibility that although you have the ability to help, you shouldn't. Newton's Third Law of Motion says, "For every action, there's an equal and opposite reaction." In the same way, there are also consequences for our actions in life. Good consequences are reinforcing—they teach us, "Hey, I want more where that came from, so I'll keep on doing what I did to get it!" while bad consequences teach us, "Well, that stunk. Better not do that again."

There's an apparent exception to this rule,

though: you can step in and shoulder the consequences for someone else's actions, and circumvent the process. Most of us will agree on a moral basis that it's not okay to steal the positive rewards of someone else's labor. But there's disagreement over whether shielding someone we love from the negative consequences of his or her poor choices is a "loving" thing to do.

Alice came to me with hot flashes, fatigue, weight gain, and IBS—the typical constellation of symptoms. But no matter how I tried, I couldn't get her to stick to the description of physical symptoms. What she wanted to talk about was how powerless she felt in her life. Her daughter-in-law manipulated and controlled her, and she didn't feel like she could stand up to her for fear of losing her son. Besides, wasn't it selfish for her to refuse to help with her grandkids just as much as her DIL wanted?

We spent most of the first visit discussing boundaries. I did give her a lab requisition to see about any physical causes of her symptoms and sent her home with a diet diary, but her real homework was to read "Boundaries" by Henry Cloud and John Townsend, and get it clear in her mind that rather than standing in the way of a real relationship, her 'no' would enable the possibility of a real relationship. Even if her DIL and perhaps her son reacted in anger, her health was suffering as a result of her poor boundaries and refusal to care for herself.

It turned out Alice did have very low hormones, hypothyroidism, and a poor diet, so we addressed all of those things. But the real turning point came when she told me, with a big grin, that at last she had set some lim-

its. Much to her surprise, they were well-received! She felt much closer to her family afterwards, she was sleeping better, her energy returned, she'd started exercising and she was losing weight. She told me how much more peaceful she felt once she'd become a peace maker, rather than a people pleaser.

What it comes down to is this. If the person you love recognizes that he has made poor choices and is sorry, then he's not as likely to make a similar choice in the future. In that case, shielding him from the consequences may be loving—as long as you want to, have the resources to do so, and haven't already bailed him out multiple times in the past!

However, if the person you love does not recognize that he has made a poor choice, by shielding him from the consequences, you are preventing him from learning from it. That's called enabling. Proverbs 19:19 says, "A hot-tempered man must pay the penalty; if you rescue him, you will have to do it again." It's best to let this kind of person reap what he sows, and learn the hard way.

Lilian had a son on drugs, who had become homeless because of his addiction. She told me that for a long time, she and her husband had done everything they could to "rescue" him—paying his rent so he wouldn't be homeless, giving him money, bringing him groceries, nagging him to clean up his life. But finally she had a frank con-

versation with a youth pastor who told her, "The only way your son is going to change, the only chance he has, is if you stop enabling him. Then he'll either crash and burn, or he'll turn around. But until now, he hasn't had to face any consequences for his behavior. He has no reason to change."

Lilian and her husband listened. She told me the one thing she insisted on doing was continuing to bring him groceries, because she couldn't bear the thought of him going hungry. But they allowed him to be homeless. They stopped giving him money. They stopped nagging.

About a year later, Lilian reported to me that her son had held a job for about six months, he was in a steady relationship, and he was paying rent!

Meanwhile, Lilian recovered her peace, and her health.

For more on all of these concepts, I highly recommend the book "Boundaries" by Henry Cloud and John Townsend.[1] I recommend it to patients all the time!

Emotional Freedom

Saying what you mean and understanding that it is not your responsibility to bear the consequences of another's actions will go far in preventing a situation of powerlessness. Sometimes, despite our efforts to create and sustain balance with boundaries and personal responsibility, we end up in a relationship that simply feels as if it will suck the life right out of us. These energy drainers can come in the form of difficult people or of unwanted circumstances. When faced with an energy drainer, there are essentially three ways you can respond: you can change the situation; you can change yourself so that the situation becomes tolerable; or you can leave the situation.

It takes wisdom to identify which of the three is appropriate. It's never possible to change another person (and if you try, you're almost guaranteed to make the problem worse). But you might be able to set limits on a person, by saying, "If you continue to speak to me harshly, I will not continue to associate with you." This does not change the other person; she can continue to be rude if she likes, but you won't be around to hear it. In that case, you have changed the situation. And this is not selfish: remember, we are not responsible for another person's needs, desires, or feelings. We can help as we want to and as we are able, but ultimately the needs, desires, and feelings of others are all their responsibility.

If you aren't in a position to set limits, consider re-framing the way you view the situation. Maybe the inefficiency of your coworkers becomes an opportunity for you to exercise patience. Maybe you can de-escalate a conflict by deciding to stay calm, rather than reacting with anger. We don't have control over other people, and we don't always have control over our circumstances, but we do have control over ourselves.

There are times when it's appropriate to cut your losses, though. Abuse of any kind is never acceptable, but it takes support from others to leave a toxic relationship, to walk away from an overly demanding job, or to withdraw from an important person. You definitely need spiritual and emotional support in order to make such a major change in your life, so make sure you find a good support group of friends, family, or other like-minded people who will be there for you through difficult times.

Stop and Evaluate

If you constantly feel worn out, I'd highly encourage you to identify the energy drainers in your life. Sit down in a quiet place with a pen and paper and write out your sources of stress. When you identify the biggest one or the biggest several, see which of the three approaches (change the situation, change yourself, or leave) is most appropriate. Cultivate the support you need to keep you accountable and help you through (including a qualified counselor if you feel that is necessary)… and then take the steps you need to take to help you regain power over your life.

Unfortunately, sometimes life is just stressful, and there's nothing you can do about it. In those situations, all we can do is take good care of ourselves and learn good stress management techniques.

For a quick run-down of options, I highly recommend beginning a spiritual practice if you do not have one already. Prayer has a way of grounding us, and reminding us that even though we may not be in control of a situation, there is One who is in control, and who is on our side. Journaling also really helps to get some of those spinning thoughts down on paper, and to make sense of your emotions—often this alone functions as an excellent stress management technique! I also love meditation, yoga, regular exercise especially in nature, and scheduling time to do things you enjoy. For more on stress management options, see Chapter 9.

But most of us tend to assume there's nothing we can do about our stress, even when that isn't the case. You just learned about identifying your energy drainers and sorting them into one of three categories: *things you can change, things you can refuse to tolerate, or things you can (or must) choose to accept.*

One of those stressors I hear about over and over in my practice is taking responsibility for other people's happiness. If you find that you are held captive by someone else's emotions, the first question to ask yourself is whether the person in question is a safe person, or an emotional vampire.

Emotional vampires are those who tend to suck you dry (pun fully intended—and no, I did not coin the term emotional vampires, but I wish I did). They may criticize, try to control or otherwise manipulate you. Sometimes your relationships with other people will suffer because of your relationship with them. If you feel responsible for the happiness of an emotional vampire, this kind of stressor needs to fall under the category of "things you refuse to tolerate." Nobody can force you to accept poor treatment, and nobody can emotionally manipulate you without your consent. If the relationship is unavoidable, then drawing firm and appropriate boundaries with that person is absolutely essential. Remember that *what you put up with, you end up with.*

Safe people, on the other hand, are accepting, forgiving, kind, honest, and help you to become your best self. They are "for" you. Nobody can be this way 100% of the time, of course, because we're all human—but if you tend to feel responsible for the emotions of a generally safe individual, then this falls under the category of "things you can change"— about yourself.

If you're a people pleaser, you probably don't feel right when you think someone is mad at you. That's normal—nobody likes it when someone is upset with them. And it is important that we strive to live at peace with others, so far as it depends upon us (Romans 12:18). The appropriate way to deal with a legitimate breach in a relationship is to approach the other person directly and have a conversation about it. Safe people will welcome honesty and directness, and most likely this approach will strengthen the relationship.

But if you're always thinking people are upset with you even when they're not, or if you find that your emotional well-being is contingent upon someone else's happiness, that's called codependency. Codependency is taking responsibility for something that is rightfully another person's problem, or allowing someone else to take responsibility for something that is rightfully yours.

Remember that control and responsibility go together: if it's under your control, it's probably your responsibility. If it's not under your control, then it would be pretty ridiculous to hold you responsible for it. Specifically, *your needs, desires, and feelings are your responsibility, while the needs, desires, and feelings of others are theirs.*

One important note here: even if you can give the other person what they want and you think this will make them happy, it is not your responsibility to do so.

Remember to stand your ground. If the other person doesn't like it, it's not your problem—it's theirs!

For more emotionally healthy individuals, simply identifying your destructive patterns may be enough to help you conquer them. But if you have a trauma history, you may require professional counseling to help unravel codependent tendencies. Either way, recognizing the pattern is a huge first step towards emotional freedom and healthy relationships. Attaining both is beneficial not only for your mental health, but also for your physical health and may ultimately have an impact on your longevity.

The Surprising Benefit of Healthy Relationships

Longevity researchers have discovered that, in general, centenarians are often described as likable. Perhaps this has something to do with the fact that happiness is contagious.[2] We like to be around people who are happy because they make us happy too. As a result, these happy, likable centenarians, who are genuinely compassionate and interested in other people, are relationship experts. They tend to get better care from their caregivers and also have a greater social support system, the importance of which cannot be overestimated.

In Malcolm Gladwell's book *Outliers,* he highlights the concentration of centenarians in the little

Italian immigrant community of Roseto, Pennsylvania in 1961. The community had rates of heart disease half that of the national average at the time, and nearly zero for men under 65—as well as a death rate 30-35% lower than the national average for all causes.[3] A professor of the University of Oklahoma Medical School wanted to find out why. To his surprise, he discovered that the people of Roseto had a diet that was far from healthy, they got very little exercise, and their Italian relatives back in Italy enjoyed no similar protection (so they didn't have their genes to thank). But something else also set them apart from the national norm: community living and multi-generational homes. Neighbors strolled the streets together in the evenings. They went to church together. They had dinner together. Their children played together. They looked out for each other.

A generation later, the "old ways" began to change as the younger generation in Roseto grew up and moved away, and the very close-knit community life the immigrants had enjoyed began to disintegrate. Over the next decade, heart disease in Roseto doubled, hypertension tripled, and the rate of fatal heart attacks reached the national average by the end of the 1970s.

It turned out that what kept that idyllic community healthy was the community itself.

* * *

The Take-Home Message:

Healthy relationships are important—not only for your quality of life, but also for your health. If you're not already plugged into a community, make it a priority to seek one out. Find a community of like-minded individuals. A great place to try out is a church, and particularly a small group or a Bible study within a church. These groups are small enough that it's still possible to get to know people within them, and they share a common faith to bring them together. Churches are excellent places to find those whose desire is to "do life together."

Another option I love is meetup.com. You can search on this website for any hobby you happen to fancy, and find groups near you of other individuals who share your interest—from hiking to knitting to philosophy discussions to ethnic cuisine. Sign up to receive emails of when and where they plan to meet next. If you can't find a meetup group that matches your interest, you can start one! Anyone who has indicated an interest in the keywords you use to describe your group will receive an email alert that the group has been created, and an invitation to join.

Why not try volunteering? Nothing helps us to feel so fulfilled as serving others in need. More on this in the next chapter!

You also might consider taking a continuing education class. Remember college—how easy it was to just meet your classmates and form study groups that turned into friendships? This might be a way to recreate that. If you're older and you're looking at a local university or community college for this, you probably would want to make sure that the course you chose was listed as "continuing education" or "non-degree seeking," to make it more likely that there might be others in a similar life stage to yours among the students.

CHAPTER 9

Building Block #9: Peace and a Sense of Purpose

According to psychologist Abraham Maslow, mankind attempts to meet his needs in a particular hierarchy. First, he will meet his physiological needs—those functions necessary for immediate survival. Once those needs have been attended to, he will meet his need for security, ensuring that his survival needs will be met for the future. After that, he will meet his need for community—that is, love and friendship. Then he will attend to his self-perception, including achievement of personal goals and respect from others.

But even once these needs are met, the final crowning desire is for self-actualization, or reaching his highest potential.[1] According to the author of the biblical Proverbs (27:20), no one ever fully realizes it in this life, and this is as it must be: consider the men who walked on the moon or won Olympic golds and then fell into despair after the fact, having nothing higher to achieve. The point is the process. So, if you've climbed Maslow's ladder and currently linger somewhere between self-perception and self-actualization, what comes next?

Finding Purpose

I found nuggets of wisdom addressing this question in Timothy Ferriss's *The Four Hour Work Week.* [2] Assuming you have the luxury of time to devote to this question, this is what he has to say on the subject (in no particular order):

First do nothing. This is absolutely necessary, because modern life is loud. If we want to hear anything other than external noise, we have to choose it consciously. The purpose of this is to tune in, and learn to make the distinction between your inner voice and the opinions and ideas of the world around you. Be warned, though: this is scary. Silence has a way of bringing up deep questions and fears. If silence is completely out of your comfort zone, just start with a few minutes per day of breathing quietly and tuning in, expanding the length of time gradually as you become more comfortable with the process.

Personal story here: during one of my quarter breaks in medical school, I decided to take my own five day fasting and meditation retreat, even though I didn't go anywhere. The goal was to really get quiet before God and tune in to whatever He might be trying to communicate to me. I watched no TV or movies, I didn't schedule any social activities, and I didn't read any books except scripture. I journaled, and I got out into nature... a lot.

It was HARD. I started going stir-crazy within the first 12 hours. I got depressed, and found it almost impossible to focus my mind on any one thing for any length of time. I started to realize that I was essentially going through withdrawal from the constant activity and stimuli in my life.

By about the third day, the restlessness passed. Nothing extraordinary happened on the other end of that retreat externally—but I can say that some key areas in my mindset shifted. My trust in God deepened. My purpose didn't exactly solidify, but it grew much clearer than it had been before. I also learned how loud my life was, and how distracted I had been as a baseline. I've been able to carry that awareness forward, checking in with myself at various points to see if I'm becoming distracted and unfocused, and attempting to realign myself with where I want to be.

Recognize that we are designed to problem-solve. Even when our lives are going well for the most part, left to our own devices, we all have a tendency to focus on what still needs fixing. Don't beat yourself up about it, but don't become a victim either. In his book, *Learned Optimism,* Martin Seligman describes a cohort of clinically depressed patients whose only treatment was a daily gratitude journal, which served to shift their focus from the problems still to be solved to the blessings that had been solved already. The result? Ninety-four percent of them reported subjective improvement in their depressive symptoms within a month.[3] The point is, when you get quiet, your mind will naturally gravitate towards the problems in your life. Be conscious of this and redirect those thoughts.

Choose an ambitious goal. The answer to fulfillment is bigger than just gratitude: if we learn to appreciate where we are, all we've done is override the natural bent of of our minds to (as Ferriss writes) "turn inward on itself and create problems for us to solve, even if the problems are undefined or unimportant." The solution he proposes is to choose some seemingly impossible goal that resonates with us. Once we've identified the goal, we start moving towards it. Now our focus is "out there." We are energized and focused. We have purpose. Most of the time when we talk about such elusive concepts as "self-esteem," this is what we're really discussing. The word self-esteem can be misleading, though, because purpose usually resides outside of ourselves. It has to do with how we can contribute to the well-being of others, how we can make the world a better place, or how we can help to support and care for those we love.

In Viktor Frankl's book, *Man's Search for Meaning,* the Jewish psychiatrist who survived the concentration camps writes, "This uniqueness and singleness which distinguishes each individual and gives a meaning to his existence has a bearing on creative work as much as it does on human love. When the impossibility of replacing a person is realized, it allows the responsibility which a man has for his existence and its continuance to appear in all its magnitude. A man who becomes conscious of the responsibility he bears toward a human being who affectionately waits for him, or to an unfinished work, will never be able to throw away his life. He knows the 'why' for his existence, and will be able to bear almost any 'how.'" According to Frankl, the pursuit of happiness is the wrong focus; happiness results from having and fulfilling one's purpose. Or to quote Frankl again, "What man actually needs is not a tensionless state but rather a striving and struggling for a worthwhile goal, a freely chosen task." [4]

Obviously, having a purpose is imperative, but you may have more than one single purpose. I've always wondered what happens to the hero of an adventure story after the story ends... if the quest consumed his whole life, his prospects after the fact seem pretty bleak. It is very common for people whose jobs or parenthood largely define them to suffer from depression after retirement, or when the kids leave home. But remember.... if you're still here, you still have more to do. How many things are on your 'bucket list'? How many causes are you passionate about? How many talents have you yet to fully develop? If you cannot answer these questions, start with step one... get quiet. Do nothing, stick with it, and wait for the answers to come.

Take Inventory

Part of waiting for the answers to come is to stop and take inventory of your life. How's it working out for you? Are you happy with not only where you are now, but with where you are headed in the major areas of your life (your relationships, your finances, your job, and your health — all aspects of it)?

If not, here's a exercise, called the One Page Miracle (I borrowed this from Dr. Amen, author of

Change Your Brain, Change Your Life).[5] It goes like this:

Separate your life into those four major categories (Relationships, Work, Money, Myself). Then break each category down further into subcategories.

For example, under relationships, if you are married, put spouse/partner, as well as children if you have them, extended family, and friends. Then write down a specific, measurable goal for the next year in each of those subcategories. (For instance, "I would like to call my adult children once a week," or "I would like to plan and schedule a date night with my husband once a week.") Here's your template:

RELATIONSHIPS
- **Spouse/Partner:**
- **Children:**
- **Extended Family:**
- **Friends:**

"Work" is whatever you spend most of your time doing. If you are a stay-at-home mom, then it will overlap with the relationship section, but it will include things like teaching your children how to play well with others, and planning time to shower every day while they're napping (I know that can be a challenge sometimes!) If you have multiple jobs, or a job and an important hobby, that goes here too. If you volunteer, that goes here. Again, make sure what you write down is specific, actionable, and measurable

—"what gets measured gets improved," after all.

WORK
- **My job:**
- **My hobby:**
- **Volunteering:**

"Money" should be broken down into short term and long term goals. I recommend breaking the short term goal down to a fiscal quarter (three months) while the long-term goal should be more where you'd like to be financially within the next year. If you're in debt, perhaps the goal could be to pay down a certain amount of your credit card bill each month, and put a certain amount in savings.

MONEY
- **Short term:**
- **Long term:**

Under "myself", you should include body, mind, and spirit, since we are comprised of all three. Most people's goals tend to focus only on the first, but true health means all of the above, and is heavily influenced by the quality of our relationships, work, and finances. It's impossible to be truly healthy without maintaining order in all of those categories.

So for your body, consider resolutions to eat healthier, exercise more, drink more water, take your vitamins, and get enough sleep… as well as perhaps to minimize any health-related addiction you may battle (alcohol, soda, smoking, overeating, too much sugar, etc). This latter point may require accountability from others to keep you honest.

Let's lump thoughts and emotions together under 'mind.' These goals may include cultivating a positive body image (especially as a counterbalance to some of the weight-loss goals in the body category), finding and pursuing a new interest to keep you intellectually stimulated, being kinder to yourself, playing more, or eliminating your "energy suckers."

And spirit involves connection with a higher power. I have certainly found that many "energy suckers" in the mind category must be dealt with on a spiritual level. A solid belief in a God who cares for you and acts positively on your behalf is a critical ingredient for deep healing from old wounds and getting out of our own way on the road to happiness and fulfillment. If you don't have a spiritual belief system or practice that is meaningful and important to your life, this is the time to start.

MYSELF
- **Body:**

- **Mind:**
- **Spirit:**

All of this should fit into a single page so that it's simple, direct, and actionable. In order for this exercise to be as effective as possible, keep your page in a place where you can see it every day. This will remind you going forward to make choices in keeping with your goals, and will make it much more likely that you will actually achieve them.

Dealing With Indecision

You may find yourself struggling with indecision when making some of the choices that will put you on the path to achieving your goals. This indecision is one of our biggest sources of stress and anxiety. I developed my approach to this one for myself originally (I definitely have this problem!), and now I share it with my patients. It's a step-wise process, based on biblical teaching, and it goes like this.

Give it to God

The first step is to realize that you are not in control anyway—that is an illusion. Think back over the events in your life: list the other times that you have tried to control your circumstances.

Did it work? What was the outcome?

Most of the time, if we're honest, we know that the answer to this is no. Sometimes we think we're in control, but we all have plenty of stories in our lives that prove this isn't ultimately the case. Admit that you are powerless to make your life work out the way you want it to. As long as you're in denial about that, you'll stay stuck.

- "Unless the Lord builds the house, its builders labor in vain. Unless the Lord watches over the city, the watchmen stand guard in vain" (Psalm 127:1).
- "There is no wisdom, no insight, no plan that can succeed against the Lord" (Proverbs 21:30).
- "Many are the plans in a man's heart, but it is the Lord's purpose that prevails" (Proverbs 19:21).
- "In his heart a man plans his course, but the Lord determines his steps" (Proverbs 16:9)

After you realize that you are not in control, acknowledge that God wants to be first in your life. This is the key to defeating control and anxiety: we are anxious when we want something more than we want to follow God. Letting go of the thing we desire is terrifying (in fact, it feels a lot like dying to ourselves), but it is the only path to peace. The paradox is, God promises that if we lose our life, that is when we will find it. As long as we insist on controlling our lives, it will remain forever out of control.

- "Seek first his kingdom and his righteousness, and all these things will be given to you as well. Therefore do not worry about tomorrow, for tomorrow will worry about itself. Each day has enough trouble of its own" (Matthew 6:33-34).
- "Whoever pursues righteousness and love finds life, prosperity and honor" (Proverbs 21:21).
- "Whoever finds their life will lose it, and whoever loses their life for my sake will find it" (Matthew 10:39).
- "For whoever wants to save their life will lose it, but whoever loses their life for me will find it" (Matthew 16:25).
- "Delight yourself in the Lord and he will give you the desires of your heart" (Psalm 37:4).
- "Blessed are the poor in spirit, for theirs is the kingdom of heaven" (Matthew 5:3).
- "Blessed are the meek, for they will inherit the earth" (Matthew 5:5).

When we let go of "trying to find our lives" (whatever the problem is that obsesses us), we will experience grief—but it is a good, healing grief. It is a grief that leads to joy in the end, because it is the only path to life.

• "Those who sow in tears will reap with songs of joy" (Psalm 126:5).

• "Blessed are those who mourn, for they will be comforted" (Matthew 5:4).

• "Weeping may remain for a night, but rejoicing comes in the morning" (Psalm 30:5).

You must know that while you are experiencing grief, you do not have to bear your pain alone. **God invites you to bring your troubles to Him.** Read his words to remind yourself that he will comfort you:

• "Come to me, all you who are weary and burdened, and I will give you rest" (Matthew 11:28).

• "Cast all your anxiety on him because he cares for you" (1 Peter 5:7).

• "Do not be anxious about anything, but in everything, by prayer and petition, with thanksgiving, present your requests to God. And the peace of God, which transcends all understanding, will guard your hearts and your minds in Christ Jesus" (Philippians 4:4-7).

• "Cast your cares on the Lord and he will sustain you; He will never let the righteous fall" (Psalm 55:22).

God is a good God; therefore you can trust Him. He is for you and not against you; He wants

good things for you. If you have trouble remember-
ing this, read over the following verses:

- "You whom I have upheld since you were
conceived, and have carried since your birth. Even to
your old age and gray hairs I am he, I am he who will
sustain you. I have made you and I will carry you; I
will sustain you and I will rescue you" (Isaiah
46:3-4).

- "I will rejoice in doing them good and will
assuredly plant them in this land with all my heart
and soul" (Jeremiah 33:41).

- "The Lord is good, a stronghold in the day of
trouble; and he knoweth them that trust in
him" (Nahum 1:7).

- "And the Lord will guide you continually and
satisfy your desire in scorched places and make your
bones strong; and you shall be like a watered garden,
like a spring of water, whose waters do not fail" (Isaiah 58:11).

- "Those who seek the Lord lack no good
thing" (Psalm 34:10).

- "For the Lord God is a sun and shield; The
Lord bestows favor and honor; No good thing does
he withhold From those whose walk is
blameless" (Psalm 84:11).

- "Praise the Lord, O my soul, And forget not
all his benefits—Who forgives all your sins And

heals all your diseases, Who redeems your life from the pit And crowns you with love and compassion, Who satisfies your desires with good things So that your youth is renewed like the eagle's" (Psalm 103:2-5).

• "You open your hand and satisfy the desires of every living thing. …He fulfills the desires of those who fear him" (Psalm 145:16-19).

Once you have brought your troubles to God, and prayed for a solution, your job is to do the very hardest thing of all: **wait, and trust that God will do what He said He would do.**

• "Wait on the Lord: be of good courage, and he shall strengthen thine heart: wait, I say, on the Lord" (Psalm 27:14).

• "Trust in the Lord, and do good; so shalt thou dwell in the land, and verily thou shalt be fed. Delight thyself in the Lord; and he shall give thee the desires of thine heart. Commit thy way unto the Lord; trust also in him; and he shall bring it to pass" (Psalm 37:3-5).

• "Trust in the Lord with all your heart and lean not on your own understanding; in all your ways acknowledge him and he will make your paths straight" (Proverbs 3:5-6).

• "You will keep in perfect peace him whose

mind is steadfast, because he trusts in you" (Isaiah 26:3).

• "Yet the Lord longs to be gracious to you; he rises to show you compassion. For the Lord is a God of justice. Blessed are all who wait for him!" (Isaiah 30:18)

• "I will repay you for the years the locusts have eaten" (Joel 2:25).

• "Will he not bring to fruition my salvation and grant me my every desire?" (2 Samuel 23:5)

• "Every good and perfect gift is from above, coming down from the Father of heavenly lights, who does not change like shifting shadows" (James 1:17).

But what if you are still supposed to do something to fix the problem? Part of trusting God is trusting that **He will tell you what to do and when to do it (if you are supposed to do anything at all).** That is why we have the Holy Spirit—he promises to guide you into all truth.

• "But the Counselor, the Holy Spirit, whom the Father will send in my name, will teach you all things and will remind you of everything I have said to you" (John 14:26).

• "But when he, the Spirit of truth, comes, he will guide you into all truth. He will not speak on his own; he will speak only what he hears, and he will tell you what is yet to come" (John 16:13).

- "Call unto Me and I will show thee great things and difficult, which thou knowest not" (Jeremiah 33:3).
- "This is what the Lord says: 'Stand at the crossroads and look; ask for the ancient paths, ask where the good way is, and walk in it, and you will find rest for your souls'" (Jeremiah 6:16).
- "I will instruct you and teach you in the way you should go; I will counsel you and watch over you" (Psalm 32:8).
- "And he will teach us of his ways, and we will walk in his paths" (Isaiah 2:3).
- "If any of you lacks wisdom, he should ask God, who gives generously to all without finding fault, and it will be given to him. But when he asks, he must believe and not doubt, because he who doubts is like a wave of the sea, blown and tossed by the wind. That man should not think he will receive anything from the Lord; he is a double-minded man, unstable in all he does" (James 1:5-8).
- "Whether you turn to the right or to the left, your ears will hear a voice behind you, saying, "This is the way; walk in it" (Isaiah 30:21).
- "Who, then, is the man that fears the Lord? He will instruct him in the way chosen for him. He

will spend his days in prosperity, and his descendants will inherit the land" (Psalm 25:12-13).

When you act according to the leading of the Holy Spirit, now you are partnering with God and can have faith in the outcome. The Bible defines faith as "the substance of things hoped for; the evidence of things not seen" (Hebrews 11:1). There's a reason why it is called substance and evidence. Hope is not the same thing as faith; hope is simply a wish or desire, while faith is the belief that that wish will come to pass. You've got to have a reason for faith (while you need none for hope). Faith is the substantive evidence of something that does not yet have physical form.

• "And the Lord will guide you continually and satisfy your desire in scorched places and make your bones strong; and you shall be like a watered garden, like a spring of water, whose waters do not fail" (Isaiah 58:11).

• "It is God who works in you to will and to act according to his good purpose" (Philippians 2:13).

• "I am the Lord your God, who teaches you what is best for you, who directs you in the way you should go" (Isaiah 48:17).

• "By his power he may fulfill every good purpose of yours and every act prompted by your faith" (2 Thessalonians 1:11).

The Enemy of Faith: Fear

If you do not have faith, you will have fear. Fear is the substance of things *dreaded*. There is a great deal of power in what you think—not because of metaphysics, but because thoughts become words, and words become actions, and actions bear consequences in our lives, whether good or bad.

Fear has a purpose: it's there to signal impending danger and to warn us to be careful. But it can be blown out of proportion to the actual danger. This is in part because the prefrontal cortex of the human brain is designed to simulate an experience before it happens. This keeps us from having to learn every lesson by hard knocks... but if we choose to imagine every possible negative scenario, no matter how unlikely, then our fear response can be very much exaggerated.

One thing that leads to fear is overgeneralization: we take a single negative event and assume that event will become a pattern. For instance, after a breakup, we conclude, "No one will ever want me. I'll be alone forever." This can become a self-fulfilling prophecy, affecting our choices and the opportunities to which we avail ourselves. (If you think no one will ever want you, how much confidence do you think you're going to give off?)

Labeling also leads to fear: we take a single negative action and generalize it to the person who committed it—ourselves or someone else. For instance, after getting fired, we conclude, "I'm a failure." Or, your spouse does something to hurt you and you conclude, "He is a selfish person." This, too, can become a self-fulfilling prophecy: if you treat someone as selfish, he's less likely to be kind to you in the future. If you tell yourself you're a failure, what are the chances you'll take any risks that might lead to success?

Worst-Case-Scenario Thinking: Pessimists usually say that life has taught them to expect the worst. They think they are protecting themselves from disappointment, no matter how unlikely their predictions might be. Proverbs 4:23 says, "Above all else, guard your heart, for it is the wellspring of life." This is because, in reality, pessimists are flooding their bodies with fight-or flight stress hormones, which, over time, can lead to high blood pressure, high cholesterol, heart disease, diabetes, insomnia, sexual dysfunction, anxiety, constipation, diarrhea, immune dysfunction, depression, and even cancer. All this, when more often than not, the things we fear don't even happen!

Fear is a kind of bondage. It is essentially meditation upon something negative instead of upon something positive, which eventually leads to the belief that a negative event will come to pass. If you find that negative thoughts regularly cloud your mind (and your mood), work on recognizing them as they pop up so that you can take a breath, acknowledge the thought, and then release it. Those thoughts do not need to take up residence in your mind. If you find that you have difficulty with this—and most people do—I encourage you to begin a meditation practice.

Mindfulness

There are a surprising number of studies that demonstrate the health benefits of meditation—just go to www.pubmed.com, type in meditation, and you'll see what I mean. Even in the mainstream arena, mindfulness is catching on as an excellent way to moderate stress.[6]

Meditation and an attitude of mindfulness melt away stress as you learn to reacquaint yourself with the richness of life's details that have gradually begun to escape your notice—your breath, the way your body feels, the beauty and movement of the plants outside, or the breeze across your skin.

Start slowly and for a short time. For five minutes, count your breaths up to eight and down again, and allow thoughts to come and go as they may, without fighting them. As you realize you are having a thought, let it go and gently redirect your thoughts back to your breath. Don't beat yourself up: it'll be hard at first, and you'll probably have a lot of thoughts fighting for your attention. But it will get easier over time.

The Take-Home Message:

- **Take inventory**. What are your goals in the major areas of your life: in your relationships, your work, your finances, and your personal growth? Do you feel as if you have a clear purpose, or a set of purposes? If not, get quiet—avoid the external stimuli, get through the withdrawals, and wait for the answers to come.
- **Start meditating**. Getting quiet once is not enough; it needs to become a lifestyle. You can't just set your life course and then expect to reach it without constant course corrections along the way—and

one of the blessings of frequent meditations or quiet periods is that it will allow you to recognize when you have gotten off course.

• **Pay attention to your thoughts**. When you are not specifically setting aside time to meditate, you're probably still "meditating," or ruminating, or something. Make sure that thing is both true, and beneficial for you. More on this in Chapter 18.

Part 3:

Obstacles to Cure

CHAPTER 10

Obstacle to Cure #1: Toxic Buildup from Food

Before I start delving into various different obstacles to cure, let me start by saying this is not designed to induce fear, but rather to promote awareness, and allow you to become conscious of what you are putting into your body so that you can make better choices.

That said: instead of food, most of the things we eat could more appropriately be called "food-like products." Experts now estimate that diet alone is responsible 30-35% of cancer cases,[1] and that's to say nothing of all of the diet-related autoimmune disorders, gut microbiota imbalances, acute poisonings or nutrient deficiencies, and all of their related manifestations.

You have control over what you put into your mouth, so that means you can take some of the responsibility for your future health. The first thing you need to learn about to do this is how to identify fake food. It is actually very simple to recognize once you know what to look for. The second lesson on food, however, can be a little trickier, because there are a number of foods available that have what seem to be decent ingredients, but are actually harmful. You'll learn to recognize those too.

There are a few easy ways to identify fake food: *if it is something that your grandparents wouldn't have recognized* or *it comes in a package,* there is a pretty good chance it is not real food. We live in a busy world, though, and I know walking away from quick-to-prepare meals is nearly impossible for some families. That means you'll have to learn how to read labels.

To start with, look for chemical additives. A quick rule of thumb is, if you can't pronounce it, don't eat it. But here are some of the specifics.

Artificial Food Colors

Artificial food colors are an obvious place to start. They are nearly everywhere, and with the petroleum-based FD&C (approved for food, drug, and cosmetic use) colors, often easy to see. These are the colors you associate with candy, brightly colored breakfast cereals, fruit-flavored sodas, rainbow colored frozen treats and baked goods. FD&C colors are also found in places that you wouldn't necessarily think to look, like fruit snacks and fruit paste products (think bars, tarts, and pies), gelatin desserts, cheeses in all of their forms, sausages, salad dressings, spice mixes, flavored yogurts, frozen meals, and even lemonades. You will be able to recognize these food dyes easily by their names: Blue No. 1 and Blue No. 2, Green No. 3, Red No. 3, Red No. 40, Yellow No. 5, and Yellow No. 6. Collectively these are associated with allergies, brain tumors, bladder and testicular cancer, thyroid tumors, adrenal tumors, kidney tumors, and ADD/ADHD, as well as hypersensitivity reactions.[2] For these reasons and more, food dyes are banned in Norway and Austria, and contain warnings in the UK and the EU. Those countries use natural food dyes such as beet juice, beta-carotene, blueberry juice concentrate, carrot juice, grape skin extract, paprika, purple sweet potato or corn, red cabbage, and turmeric.

You can pretty well assume that anything derived from petroleum (i.e. crude oil, also found in gasoline, asphalt, and tar) shouldn't go in your mouth. But just in case you need convincing to stop buying your child's favorite products, let's look at each synthetic color individually:

- **Blue #1** has been shown to trigger allergies. (And is that any wonder? The immune system mounts an allergic response to unknown invaders, just in case they might be pathogenic. Food dyes are petrochemicals; they're not food. It makes sense that the body would want to guard against them, doesn't it?)
- **Blue #2** is associated with brain cancer.
- **Green #3** has been associated with thyroid cancer.
- **Red #3** has been recognized by the FDA (Food and Drug Administration) as a carcinogen (cancer-causing substance) for years.
- **Red #40** is commonly contaminated with known carcinogens and is known to cause allergic reactions.
- **Yellow #5** (tartrazine) is especially linked with childhood behavior problems and causes the type of hyperactivity that is typically associated with ADD/ADHD. (If your kid has ADD/ADHD, get them off food dyes ASAP!) On top of that, Yellow #5 is also a known allergen and is routinely contaminated with carcinogens.
- **Yellow #6** is yet another allergenic carcino-

gen and has been associated, in particular, with kidney cancer.

Unfortunately, our list of artificial colors doesn't end there. There is another color you need to be aware of; it is found just as often in "natural" products as in the mainstream brands and the amounts and types of products it is put into is staggering. This ubiquitous carcinogen (remember, that means it causes cancer) is Caramel Coloring.[3] Caramel Coloring is found in colas, soy and Worcestershire sauces, chocolate-flavored products, beer, and pre-cooked meats, to name just a few items. Again, it is often referred to as natural because it is a sugar-based product, but do not be fooled. Caramel Coloring is produced by heating sugar with ammonia or ammonium compounds (you don't cook with ammonia at home, do you?)

Artificial colors can directly impact our health, but there is another reason they should be avoided: they convince people to eat processed junk instead of real food, because they dress up the food-like product to make it appear more enticing. You can bet any food product containing artificial coloring contains a host of other chemicals as well, and chances are it's been stripped of any real nutritional value too. Do we really want to entice people to eat more of that crap?

Preservatives

Preservatives are commonly included in processed foods to increase shelf life. They have been associated with allergic reactions and are stored in body fat (which means it's hard to get rid of them). While you are reading labels, make sure to avoid:

• **BHA** (Butylated hydroxyanisole) and **BHT** (Butylated hydroxytoluene): These are found in prepared and packaged foods where they are used as a preservative for fat. They have been linked with cancer in rats, mice, and hamsters (so, for good reason, it's a suspected carcinogen in humans). Often these two are used with Propyl Gallate, a preservative of fats as well, also a suspected carcinogen. BHA may also induce allergic reactions and hyperactivity in some sensitive patients. BHA and BHT are banned Japan, in the UK (in infant foods), and in parts of the EU.
• **Sodium Benzoate/Benzoic Acid**: used as a preservative in juices, sodas, and pickles and found in shrimp and fish. When used in beverages containing ascorbic acid (Vitamin C), the two react to form small amounts of benzene, a known carcinogen (can-

cer-causing agent).

• **Sulfites** (sulfur dioxide, sodium bisulfite): preservatives and bleaching agents in some wine, dried fruit, and processed shrimp and potatoes, these are also sprayed on fruit, veggies, and shrimp, and are associated with asthma. Sulfites can cause severe asthma reactions in sensitive individuals and are also a relatively common trigger for migraines. (You can find all of the aforementioned foods without sulfites —just read your labels.)

• **Trans Fats, aka Partially Hydrogenated Oils**: Trans fat means that hydrogen has been added to a liquid fatty acid to render it solid at room temperature, increasing its shelf life while also improving texture or "mouth feel." It's found in margarine, shortening, fried foods, and all kinds of processed foods. Trans fats are incorporated into your cell walls, causing poor cell membrane and receptor function, and they also increase "bad" cholesterol (LDL) and lower "good" cholesterol (HDL). This contributes to a number of chronic diseases, including heart disease and cancer.[5] Trans fats also lower immune system function and increase insulin resistance. Avoid them completely if at all possible.

• **Sodium nitrate/ sodium nitrite**: The World Cancer Research Fund (WCRF) reviewed more than 7000 clinical studies investigating the links between cancer and diet choices, and concluded: "World Cancer Research Fund International recommends avoiding processed meat. This is the conclusion of an independent panel of leading scientists who, following the biggest review of international research ever undertaken, judged the evidence that processed meat increases the risk of bowel cancer to be convincing. This review was done in 2007 and was subsequently confirmed in 2011." [6] Even more compelling to me because my family history includes pancreatic cancer, a study out of the University of Hawaii in 2005 showed that consumption of processed meat products including nitrates and nitrites increased the risk of pancreatic cancer by 68%. [7] Added to preserve color and prolong shelf life, in the body these form carcinogenic (cancer-causing) nitrosamines. Nitrates and/or nitrites can be found in bacon, sausage, hot dogs, beef jerky, lunch meats, and virtually any prepackaged meal containing meat (including pepperoni and salami). The American Cancer Society further notes that high consumption of processed meat over a decade is associated with a 50% increase in the risk for bowel and rectal cancers—where "high consumption" for men is about two slices of bacon OR half a hot dog, 5-6 days per week, and for women, a similar amount 2-3 days per week. [8]

This doesn't mean you can't ever have bacon again, but you should be vigilant about the meat products you buy. Health food stores carry bacon (and sausage, and hot dogs) that do not contain nitrates or nitrates, and they'll usually advertise that they are nitrate-free on the front of the package. If not, flip it over and read the ingredients. If it lists nitrates or nitrites, put it back. You can also make your own sausage: free range ground turkey plus a little salt, pepper, sage, and cumin tastes quite similar to the prepackaged varieties! I'd recommend caution with deli meats and processed meat products purchased in restaurants, though—you can easily end up falling into the "high consumption" category if you eat out a lot. When you can opt for unprocessed meats, do so.

But if (for instance) your office caters in grinders from the deli for a lunch meeting and your choice is between eating it or going hungry, you can offset the negative impact of the nitrates and nitrites with some extra vitamin C. Ascorbic acid helps block the conversion of nitrates and nitrites to carcinogenic nitrosamines, so it can help protect you in a pinch. So choose a side dish that's rich in Vitamin C (such as broccoli, bell peppers, and citrus fruits), or keep some extra Vitamin C tablets in your purse or your desk, just in case.

* * *

Sugar Substitutes

As a general rule, even though excessive sugar is a bad idea, if you must sweeten your food, it's actually a better idea to use real sugar than the stuff created in a lab. That's because sugar alcohols and artificial sweeteners are your main alternatives.

Sugar alcohols like isomalt, lactitol, sorbitol, mannitol, and xylitol are not as sweet as sugar and often sound like a good sugar alternative because they have a much lower glycemic index and don't cause tooth decay—but the reason they have a lower glycemic index is because they are poorly absorbed. This means that they hang out longer in the gut, increasing the risk of gas and bloating, and in some cases loose stools and diarrhea. A little here and there is okay for most people, but it's probably therefore a good idea to not overdo them.

Artificial sweeteners you will find on labels are Acesulfame-potassium, Splenda/sucralose, Equal or NutraSweet/aspartame, Sweet 'N Low/saccharin. Just in case you are thinking to yourself that your one special beverage won't harm you, here are some specifics:

* **Saccharin**: an artificial sweetener found in Sweet and Low, 300-500 times sweeter than sugar.

It's associated with bladder cancer when fed to rats in large quantities.

• **Aspartame**: found in Nutrasweet and Equal. It gets metabolized to excitatory amino acids which can lead to neuronal cell death, and has been linked with various neurological diseases such as MS, ALS, and Alzheimer's Disease.[9] It has also been linked to a number of adverse food reactions including headaches, migraines, depression, seizures, weight gain, irritability, insomnia, joint pain, and memory loss.

• **Sucralose**: found in Splenda, which is 600 times sweeter than sugar. Its byproducts are in the same chemical category as certain pesticides (PCBs and DDT), and inconclusive studies suggest that it may cause genetic mutations. High doses have been linked with lower immune function.

Individual Additives

You now know the major groups (artificial colors, preservatives, sugar substitutes) of additives that need to be avoided, but there are a few more that don't fit neatly into a category and must be remembered by name.

• **Monosodium Glutamate/MSG**: used as a

flavor enhancer in various processed foods, it is especially common in Chinese food prepared in restaurants, where it is added to increase the salty flavor of protein. It is primarily a problem only for individuals who are sensitive (sensitivities include headaches and migraines, nausea, burning sensations, increased heart rate, weakness, and wheezing or difficulty breathing) or allergic (chest tightness, diarrhea, headaches, and flushing). However, large amounts have been associated with neural damage in animal studies.

- **Olestra/Olean**: These fat substitutes are found in "fat-free" chips primarily. (Note: any packaged food that boasts "fat-free," "sugar-free" or "fortified" usually makes up for it with a cocktail of chemicals. AVOID.) Like their "sugar-free" cousins, sugar alcohols, olestra manages to taste like fat without the same impact on the body because it's indigestible. Side effects therefore include diarrhea, cramps and leaky bowels, as well as poor absorption of fat soluble vitamins such as A, D, E and K. As if that wasn't bad enough, in 2011, Purdue University demonstrated that rats fed potato chips made with Olean actually gained weight. Olestra and Olean are banned in the UK and Canada.

- **Potassium Bromate**: Potassium bromate gets added to commercial bread products because it improves the volume of bread by helping the dough hold together and rise higher, and it is also approved by the FDA for use in malting barley. Bromate usually breaks down into bromide, which does not appear to be harmful. However, bromate itself is a carcinogen in animals. Some studies indicate that potassium bromate may be carcinogenic, and link it to nervous system and kidney damage. Potassium Bromate is also one of the possible contributors to the hypothyroidism epidemic (more on this in Chapter 17). Due to the location of bromine on the periodic table, it behaves very much like iodine, thus acting as a competitive inhibitor of iodine and potentially interfering with the production of thyroid hormone. It is banned in Canada, China and the EU.

• **Brominated Vegetable Oil**: BVO shows up in a number of beverages, such as Mountain Dew, Fresca, and some flavors of Powerade (though it was recently removed from Gatorade). It acts as an "emulsifier," helping to distribute the flavor and prevent layers of chemical separation. Again, bromine is linked to thyroid trouble (see Chapter 17), tremors, depression, confusion, and several kinds of cancer (according to Mayo Clinic). Brominated Vegetable Oil is banned in the EU and Japan.

• **Phosphoric Acid**: an additive in sodas that strips your body, and your bones, of essential nutrients. Phosphoric acid is added to soda to give it a "tangy" flavor, and it makes it very acidic. Your blood, however, has to maintain a very specific pH… and if you ingest something very acidic, it has to "buffer" that acidity with minerals, which it strips from your bones. This can set you up for osteoporosis and kidney stones.

Non-Toxic Additives You May Want to Watch Out For

Some food additives truly are natural and don't really carry a toxic burden. For health reasons, though, you should know about them so you can use them responsibly, or identify a possible sensitivity. These are two of the most common:

- **Caffeine**: Although a little caffeine isn't necessarily bad, too much definitely is. Caffeine doesn't directly increase adrenaline, but it does allow it to work unhindered. This can mean increased blood pressure, heart rate, palpitations, blood flow to the muscles, irritability and/or anxiety, as well as decreased blood flow to the brain.[10] This, again, can contribute to impaired concentration and focus if you overdo it. Too much caffeine can also contribute to adrenal fatigue, and weakened adrenals can lead to a whole host of problems (see Chapter 16). Depending on how exhausted you are, consuming caffeine to keep going is sort of like whipping a dead horse.

•   **Salicylates**: these are chemically similar to aspirin, and so people with allergies to aspirin may not tolerate them well. They are found in cake mixes, sodas, dried fruits and berries, gum, pudding, and ice cream, and they are also used to enhance the flavor of certain spices.

We've covered a lot, and at this point you may be wondering if there is anything you *can* eat. There is. To simplify, you can sum up almost everything we have covered as follows: **if it contains a chemical you don't recognize, do not put it in your mouth**. Your awareness of the toxic chemicals in our food supply is important! If the FDA does not ban these chemicals, it's up to us to vote with our dollars. If we stop buying fake foods full of petrochemicals, companies will eventually stop producing them. (After all, even Wal-Mart and Costco have begun to carry organic, nitrate- and nitrite-free, free range, and other healthy food products!)

Unlabeled Toxins

Once upon a time, food was fairly self-explanatory. You pretty much knew that a chicken was a chicken, vegetables were vegetables, and there was only one kind of milk to choose from—the kind that came out of a cow—unless you happened to prefer the milk of some other mammal.

But these days, things are a little more complicated. Unfortunately for consumers, there are a number of toxic food additives that you will never find on a label. In order to avoid them, it is necessary to seek out products that are organic, or that specifically state they do not contain the ingredient or contaminant in question.

Genetically Modified Organisms (GMOs) are perhaps the largest contributor to toxins in our food supply. Genetic modification in general involves taking a gene from one organism, clipping it out of that organism's genome (splicing it) and then inserting it into the genome of a different organism.

There's a lot of debate about whether or not that's a good idea. GMOs have been banned to varying degrees in the EU, the UK, Norway, Australia, New Zealand, Thailand, the Philippines, Saudi Arabia, Egypt, Algeria, Brazil, and Paraguay.

The two biggest GMO crops are soybeans (94% of the soybeans in the US are GM) and corn (88% in the US)—pretty much if you buy these in the US, they're genetically engineered unless they say otherwise. Other genetically modified crops include cotton, canola (which is made from rapeseed and technically isn't a food anyway), alfalfa, sugar beets, zucchini, and Hawaiian papaya. These foods are primarily engineered to be herbicide- and insect-resistant, so that they do not need as much pesticide applied to them as non-GM crops, and are resistant to herbicides. Here's the catch: there are no long-term human studies to determine safety of these crops, nor are there currently any being done. This is because the FDA considers them to be essentially equivalent to their non-GM counterparts. For that reason, GM foods are not required to be labeled. Most likely, you consume them daily without realizing it, especially if you eat a lot of processed food products.

Despite the official consensus that GM foods are safe for consumption, though, there is cause for caution. The crops often contain a gene from an organism called Bacillus thuringiensis, or Bt, which, when expressed, produces a toxin called glyphosate. This is the active ingredient in the insecticide called Round*up*, which kills insects by poking holes in the gut lining. That means these plants actually produce their own Round*up*! According to the EPA, glyphosate is toxic to insects only and has no effect on humans or animals. However, some data links glyphosate with birth defects, miscarriages, infertility, behavioral disorders, and even autism.[11]

Even more compelling to me as a naturopathic doctor is the fact that since the 1996 introduction of GM corn and soy into the US, inflammatory gastrointestinal disorders have been on the rise. Admittedly, correlation and causation are not the same thing. But I can verify in my practice that intestinal permeability, or so-called "leaky gut" syndrome, is strangely prevalent. (I make this diagnosis when according to blood food sensitivity tests, patients develop IgG reactions to more than twenty different foods.) I can also verify the connection between the gut and overall health.

More cause for concern with glyphosate-laden GM foods: glyphosate is a chelator, which means it binds to positively charged elements and compounds (such as trace minerals and nutrients) and doesn't let go. Plants treated with glyphosate may therefore be deficient in nutrients, and the evidence suggests they are primarily low in manganese, zinc, and iron. Although there are studies on both sides of the fence on this issue, it stands to reason that if true, animals eating nutrient deficient plants will then develop nutrient deficiencies themselves. At any rate, it is certainly the case that free-range poultry and grass fed meat are substantially higher in essential fatty acids (EFAs) than their agro industry counterparts, and I wonder now whether these issues are related.

So although the official position is that GM foods are safe, we don't know their long-term effects, and there's evidence that they may be harmful. I can attest to the fact that a cleaner diet nearly always dramatically improves my patients' health, although whether this is due to higher quality foods in general or the removal of GM foods specifically, I cannot say.

But in general, my rule is that if the jury's out on safety, avoid it. Be sure to choose organic soy and corn products, OR those that specifically say "non-GMO Project Verified" on the package. Also, avoid canola oil and cottonseed oil altogether… since, you know, they're not produced from edible plants.

Toxins in Meat

If you want to avoid GM foods completely, you will need to purchase organic meats too, because animals bred for slaughter are pretty well guaranteed to be fed the cheaper, chemically laden GM grains. Really, though, organic animal products are necessary anyway, because that is where the majority of our unlabelled toxins are hiding.

One of the chemicals found in our meat supply is Ractopamine. Ractopamine gets added to animal feed in the last few days before slaughter to promote leanness and increase muscle mass. But because the animals consume it so close to the end, as much as 20% of the drug makes its way into the meat we buy at the grocery store. And in us, ractopamine has been linked to hyperactivity, behavioral changes, and cardiovascular problems. It has been banned in the EU, Russia, mainland China & the Republic of China (Taiwan).

If you want to try to avoid Ractopamine by choosing fish or fowl instead, though, you are in for a nasty surprise.

We feed arsenic to our chickens in order to prevent parasites, bulk up and improve the color of the poultry meat, and decrease the chickens' feed consumption. The result is high levels of inorganic arsenic in the poultry we buy, which is carcinogenic (and also a well-known poison, hello?!) Arsenic, sensibly, has been banned from food products in the EU. Again, the way to avoid this is to buy your chicken organic.

Choosing fish over chicken may be no better, though, because farmed fish, in addition to possibly being fed artificial colors to make their flesh more appetizing, is notoriously high in heavy metals. The biggest offenders are tuna, mackeral, catfish, sturgeon, swordfish, and shark; and if you cannot afford to buy all your fish wild-caught, at the very least, avoid farmed Atlantic salmon.

Antibiotics and Dairy

About 70% of this nation's antibiotics are fed to dairy cattle to offset the unhealthy conditions in which they are maintained. Much of the need for antibiotics stems from inflammation in the cows' breast tissue due to treatment with the growth hormones rBGH and rBST (as well a diet of GMO grains which their stomachs cannot easily digest). rBGH and rBST are banned in Australia, New Zealand, Israel, the EU and Canada because the milk produced by cows treated with these hormones has a higher concentration of insulin-like growth factor-1 (IGF-1), which is linked to various kinds of hormonal cancers.

Fortunately, even many non-organic milk brands now proudly boast that they are rBGH and rBST-free, but if you want to discourage the overuse of antibiotics as well (and the resistant bacteria they help to create—more on this in Chapter 12), then you'll have to go organic.

Summary of Animal Contaminants

If you want to avoid these unlabelled contaminants in your animal products, you need to look specifically for the following:

- Dairy that says "No rBGH or rBST." Again, I'd encourage organic, because then you're skipping the antibiotics too… not to mention encouraging more humane treatment of the animals.
- Organic chicken, or at least free-range.
- Organic meat, or at least free-range.
- Wild-caught fish whenever possible.

Understanding Product Claims

When you start shopping for non-toxic food products, you will notice all the promises "this is natural!" or "this is heart-healthy!" Often they are packaged in green or brown, and cost considerably more that their shelf-mates. What do all of these claims mean, though? Are they really good for us? The short answer is "maybe." You will still need to do some label detective work.

- **Natural or Organic**: Natural just means the product does not include synthetic or artificial ingredients. That's good in the sense that you want to avoid consuming as many chemicals as possible, because, as you know now, many of them have been linked with a number of illnesses. Organic means the food is grown without fertilizers, insecticides, herbicides, or growth hormones according to USDA standards. Sometimes it's worth it to pay more for organic and sometimes it isn't, based on how full of pesticides the inorganic food tends to be. In general, for fresh produce, you want to buy the "dirty dozen" fruits and veggies organic, and it becomes less important for the "clean fifteen" (http://www.ewg.org/foodnews/summary/). If you buy organic across the board, you'll probably get a higher nutrient content because the soil will be richer (more on this in Chapter 3), but that gets pretty pricey, I know.

• **Lean and Extra Lean**: These terms apply to meat, poultry, and fish. Lean means there's less than 10 grams of fat, 4.5 grams or less of saturated fat, and 95 mg cholesterol per 100 grams. Extra lean means less than 5 gm fat, less than 2 grams saturated fat, and less than 95 mg cholesterol per 100 grams. It's a good idea to choose lean meats, as they decrease the risk of cancer otherwise associated with other meats. But it's most important to choose organic and free range meats if at all possible, because free range meats contain a better ratio of omega 3 to omega 6 (decreasing the risk of many inflammatory diseases), and again, organic meats do not contain growth hormones.

• **Enriched and Fortified**: Both of these terms

mean that vitamins and minerals were added to the food, but fortified means more of the nutrients naturally found in the food were added, while enriched means that vitamins and minerals that were lost during processing were added back. But don't think that the food itself is healthy just because the company added a few extra nutrients. If a food needs to be enriched in the first place, it's processed, and processing leads to a number of other problems. Also beware of the high sugar content commonly found in processed foods.

• **Heart Healthy**: This is a bit of a catch-all term, meaning the food is low in calories, whole grain, fat free, and/or made with oil instead of saturated fat. The label is usually unregulated though, so you should take it with a grain of salt… no pun intended.

• **Low Fat and Fat Free**: Low fat means three grams of fat or less per serving size. Fat free means what it sounds like: only traces of fat exist in the food or none at all. If you choose these foods because you're trying to lose weight, though, beware that fat free does NOT mean low calorie. In fact, often these foods contain a bunch of sugar, which is the worst option for weight loss.

• **Whole Grain**: This means that all three major components of the grain kernel remain in the food: bran, germ, and endosperm. The bran contains fiber and B vitamins, magnesium, phosphorus, iron and zinc. The germ contains Vitamin E, selenium, thiamine, iron, magnesium, phosphorus, zinc, and protein. The endosperm contains protein and carbohydrates. When grains are milled, they lose the bran and the germ, retaining only the protein and carbs from the endosperm. The lack of fiber in processed grains means that the remaining carbs hit your bloodstream almost immediately, and they act basically just like sugar. Additionally, the loss of the bran and germ removes most of the nutritional value of the grain. So whole grains are a much better idea than processed. However, be aware that unless the package specifically says that it is 100% whole grain, most likely it's been mixed with a processed ("enriched") version as well, in order to make the final product light and fluffy. So if it doesn't have that 100% on the label, or if you see the word "enriched" anywhere in the ingredient list, it's not really all that healthy.

- **Gluten Free**: Gluten is a protein found in the germ (see above) of wheat, rye, barley, and several other grains. Gluten intolerance and Celiac Disease are both relatively common, and especially for Celiac patients, total gluten avoidance is critical. That said, if you are not gluten sensitive, you don't really need to avoid it and eating gluten free some of the time will have no benefit. More on this in Chapter 14.

Low in Sodium

In addition to the previously listed product label claims, you will undoubtedly see a number of products advertising that they are low in sodium. Is that better for you? It's almost taken as a given that too much sodium is bad for your health, and especially your blood pressure. Before I address the truth of the claim, let's take a look at where this idea comes from.

Any living system seeks to create balance, or homeostasis. One aspect of this is electrolyte balance. Sodium is the most abundant electrolyte in the body, followed by chloride (not surprising, since in table salt they come together). Your body balances electrolyte concentrations found in different compartments by shifting around water content, because water can pass through membranes (while electrolytes can't, not without assistance). Therefore, when sodium concentration on one side of a membrane is higher than on the other, water content follows in order to balance it out. If you've just recently eaten a lot of sodium, the concentration will be higher in your bloodstream, so the water will flow out of your cell membranes and into your bloodstream to balance it out.

More water in the blood vessels —> higher blood volume —> higher blood pressure. So yes: too much sodium will spike your blood pressure.

The flip side is true too. If you've been under a lot of stress for a long period of time, in addition to fatigue that will probably hit you around 1-3 pm (see Chapter 16), you might notice that when you stand up too quickly, the room goes dark for a few seconds (called orthostatic hypotension). This is because your adrenal glands produce several hormones. One of them is of course cortisol, responsible for most of the classic symptoms of adrenal fatigue. But another is called aldosterone. Aldosterone reabsorbs sodium and exchanges it for potassium in the kidneys. Again, water follows sodium, so as you reabsorb sodium, you reabsorb water also. So if your adrenals are too tired to make enough aldosterone, you'll spill both sodium and water into your urine, and you'll likely notice that your blood pressure will go down. This means your heart will have to work extra hard to get the lower blood volume all the way up to your head when you stand up too fast. These people will some-times find that they crave salt… and for good reason. The body is trying to get that blood volume back up.

So bottom line: yes, sodium will cause your

blood volume to increase, and that will make your blood pressure go up. High sodium is also acidifying, which will lead to overworked kidneys, potential kidney stones, and osteoporosis (as mentioned more in depth in Chapter 4).

So is low sodium better than high sodium in a prepackaged food? Sure. But I wouldn't go to the other extreme and say all salt is bad for you; unprocessed sea salt on real food and in moderation is necessary (see Chapter 2). Also, again: if it *has* to say "low in sodium," you're looking at a prepackaged product that most likely is full of chemicals. So beware, and as always, read your labels.

Sweet Toxicity

According to Weston Price (a dentist who researched traditional diets around the world in the 1930s), the real culprits for Western diseases are white flour, sugar, and processed vegetable fats.[13] Traditional diets ranging from almost entirely plant based to almost entirely animal based all produced healthy populations; it was not until the Western processed foods listed above infiltrated those societies that health in Westernized countries around the world began to decline.

Do you know what counts as sugar? The

glycemic index is a measure of how quickly a particular food turns to sugar in the body. Glucose is assigned a glycemic index of 100, and everything else is assigned a number relative to that. At the top of the glycemic index list are all things white, especially processed white flour (including white bread, pancakes, and pastries), most processed white grains (including white rice, instant oatmeal, popcorn, and most cereals), and white potatoes, especially potato products (including french fries, potato chips, and instant mashed potatoes).

Think of sugar as quick energy. It can get converted into the currency your body uses for energy very quickly. But your blood can only accommodate a few tablespoons of sugar at a time. So your body tries to get rid of excess sugar from the bloodstream in order to minimize this process.

Sugar has to get inside the cells in order to get out of the blood. But it can't just rush into the cells— it has to have the "key" to get in. The key is called insulin, and it gets produced from the pancreas in response to high sugar in the bloodstream. This works great for a while… but problems come in when this cycle is repeated too often, too long. Like a drug addict needing a bigger dose to achieve the same high, the body will start to require more and more insulin to keep up with your sugar intake. Eventually, the pancreas won't be able to keep up with the demand. This leads to Insulin Resistance and Diabetes. That's the first problem with too much sugar, and it's a doozy.

Once the sugar gets inside the cells, it can't be stored in its present form—it has to be converted from "quick" energy into "potential" energy—AKA fat (or more precisely, triglycerides.) So sugar also leads to obesity. That's the second problem with too much sugar.

Other prevalent Western diseases linked to sugar consumption include cancer (and cancer cells consume sugar as energy before the rest of the body, so eating sugar will feed cancer cells), dementia and Alzheimer's disease, cardiovascular disease, IBS, and many more.[14]

Even knowing all this, many people find it hard to stop eating sugar. This is because sugar is an addiction, just like alcohol, smoking, and drugs. A research study found that sugar produces a chemical in the brain called enkephalins, which work much like opiates (including heroin, morphine, and oxycontin)—that is, they stimulate the release of dopamine.[15] Most other addictions do the same thing: dopamine is the neurotransmitter in the brain linked to pleasure and reward.

Do you use sugar and foods that act like sugar

(with a high glycemic index) to make you feel better after a bad day?

Do you crave sugar or high glycemic index foods?

Have you ever tried to avoid sugar and found that either you couldn't, or once you tasted something sweet you felt compelled to consume all of it?

Do you use sugar, and foods that act like sugar, as a reward for yourself?

If you answered yes to several of those questions, you are far from alone!

My 48 year old patient Jane came to me with 2/10 energy, barely able to function. She had brain fog, constant gas and bloating, and Lyme Disease with all its corresponding neurological symptoms. She also had hypothyroidism, insomnia, and a host of hormonal imbalances. After discussing with her a long and complex treatment plan at our first visit involving many diet and lifestyle changes, I told her that before we could start treating Lyme effectively, we'd need to deal with the probable overgrowth of candida albicans, a fungal organism that feeds primarily on sugar. The treatment protocol would involve complete avoidance of sugar for 6 weeks. Immediately Jane teared up. She told me she could handle anything else, but taking away her sugar was just too much!

Instead, we worked together to create a longer term but more manageable step-wise process so that she wouldn't feel so restricted: I told her that twice a day, she could have sugar, if she would strictly avoid it for the rest of the day. After a week it became once a day, and then a

few times per week.
  Eventually she successfully kicked the habit, which made treating her other symptoms and conditions much easier.

Soft Drinks, Soda, Pop, or "Cokes" (in the generic sense)

Sodas can be an exceptionally difficult habit to kick because they are everywhere. You pass them on curbs and in hallways, and they are offered in nearly every social setting. But regular soda consumption is definitely a bad habit. Here's why.

Regular sized sodas can have up to 50-80 grams of sugar *per can*. (Context: a regular size Snickers bar has 30 grams!) While adults get about 7% of their calories from soda, teenagers get some 13% from soda. Aside from all the other issues with massive sugar consumption, that can lead to some serious weight gain.

Childhood obesity has more than doubled in children and tripled in teens in the last 30 years. In 2010, more than 1/3 of children and teens were either overweight or obese, and Type 2 Diabetes (formerly referred to as "adult onset," heavily linked to obesity) has become increasingly frequent in teens and children as well.

High Fructose Corn Syrup, one of the most

common sweeteners in sodas, is especially nasty. While the body gets to choose whether it wants to use glucose (regular sugar) for energy or store it for future use (as fat), fructose bypasses this regulatory step and goes straight to fat. This means that it increases BMI and triglycerides, *but doesn't curb your appetite at all.* It's also six times as sweet as regular sugar—so just as with artificial sweeteners, it "spoils" your taste for good, natural food. Down the line, excess sugar also sets you up for heart disease, fatty liver disease and of course, diabetes.

Aside from the weight gain, the sugar in soda also has a possible relationship to ADHD symptoms: a huge influx of sugar requires a huge output of insulin, which then leads to an equally fast sugar crash. The resulting hypoglycemia (low blood sugar) symptoms include shakiness, irritability, low energy and attention span, and sugar craving (so it perpetuates the cycle of poor food choices).

Sugar is also the primary food for the intestinal organism candida. If you eat a lot of sugar over a long enough period of time, and/or if you also have a poor gut flora balance to begin with, you may end up with candida overgrowth, one of the symptoms of which is brain fog and poor memory and concentration. (More on this in Chapter 14).

People think they're being "good" by choosing

the diet versions, which instead include artificial sweeteners such as Splenda (sucralose), Equal or NutraSweet (aspartame), and Sweet 'N Low (saccharin). As mentioned earlier, collectively these chemicals are associated with leukemia, brain tumors, breast cancer, bladder cancer, uterine and ovarian cancer, skin cancer, immune dysfunction, DNA damage, preterm delivery, and neurological problems. Personally I'd rather be overweight and inattentive.

Unfortunately, diet sodas aren't even good for your waistline. Bizarrely enough, it turns out diet soda can still make you fat.

At first, this seems to make no sense—glucose (sugar) can get directly converted into triglycerides which get stored as fat, but artificial sweeteners cannot. It looks like the connection between your weight and artificial sweeteners has to do with your microbiome—the good probiotics in your gut.

Your Gut Flora and Your Weight

The Personalized Nutrition Project[15] is a study which (among other things) correlated artificial sweetener consumption with individual gut flora populations. The study found that after even a week of artificial sweetener consumption, the bacterial con figurations in the participants' guts had changed, and they started to demonstrate signs of insulin resistance.

In fact, another study from the Journal of the American Geriatrics Society[16] found that over a period of nine years, diet soda intake corresponded to three times the abdominal fat compared to non-diet soda drinkers.

(There's another implication here too, and that is that probiotics are a good addition to a weight loss regime.)

Artificial Sweeteners and Leptin

Another potential reason for the connection of artificial sweeteners and weight gain may be that, while sugar has calories and therefore triggers the release of the 'satiety' hormone leptin (which tells your body you're full and to stop eating), artificial sweeteners will stimulate the receptors in your tongue and your brain that say you're eating something sweet, without the caloric payload. This does two things: it trains you to crave sweeter treats (because artificial sweeteners are between 300-600 times sweeter than sugar), and it lowers the body's satiety response to sweetness. When sugar-like substances don't sustain us, our bodies adapt, lowering the release of leptin.

Beyond the pick-your-poison sweeteners, sodas are full of artificial colors (you now know these cause cancer and hyperactivity) and artificial flavors. [17] They also have toxic preservatives and sometimes, from a chemical reaction, benzene. In addition, because of their phosphoric acid content, they lead to mineral loss, osteoporosis and kidney stones.[18]

If you're looking to wean off of the soda habit, you might try health food alternative sodas such as Zevia, sweetened with natural stevia, or better yet, switch to unsweetened iced tea or fruit juice (which you can dilute with carbonated water if you're craving the fizz), diluting it more and more over time to cut the excess sugar. Or you can choose my favorite, and go straight for flavored carbonated water (I love the Trader Joe's brand).

Eating for Health

If you are wondering if there is anything left to eat or drink, just take a breath and know that eating healthy really isn't that hard—most of our ancestors had it figured out! If you feel overwhelmed at the store, try to remember these simple rules and it will neatly cover most of what we have discussed.

- The shorter the ingredient list, the better.

• If you don't recognize the ingredient, it doesn't go in your body if you can help it.

• Choose foods that will spoil, and eat them before they do. The less processed, the better.

• Avoid sugary, processed beverages. Especially avoid sugary, processed beverages laden with carcinogenic chemicals and food dyes.

Above all, remember that what you choose to feed your family does make a difference!

CHAPTER 11

Obstacle to Cure #2: Toxic Buildup from Personal Care Products, Mold, or other Chemicals

Our bodies are overwhelmed by the assault of chemicals in modern living. Our food, furnishings, housing, cosmetics, cleaning products, paper products, cars, and all other belongings carry the stamp of the chemical industry. I won't argue that these products are inherently bad, because they have allowed us to live in comfort and accomplish great things. But for many of us, our bodies are simply not up to the task of filtering extreme levels of novel pollutants.

Many of these toxic exposures happen either in our own homes, or because we choose products and services that are harmful to us. By understanding the dangers of everyday items and seeking appropriate substitutes, you will be able to avoid the things that don't have a risk:benefit ratio that you are comfortable with.

Endocrine Disrupting Chemicals

By far the most common illness-inducing pollutants are endocrine disrupting chemicals. They are *everywhere* and the manufacturers of those chemicals churn out millions of gallons every day.

Endocrine disrupting chemicals can screw up your hormones. Many of them are estrogenic, and the vast majority of female endocrine issues I've seen stem from estrogen dominance relative to progesterone (see Chapter 17). Quite a few of these also disrupt the thyroid, which makes sense—hypothyroidism has swelled to near-epidemic proportions as well. It is important to learn where these chemicals are hiding, because they are never advertised.

You have probably heard of the chemical **Bisphenol A (BPA)** and how the FDA has banned inclusion of BPA in baby bottles, but you may not be aware that the current FDA position is that BPA is safe. BPA is used in hard plastics and in the resin lining the insides of most food and beverage cans, and the FDA continues to hold that the BPA lining food and beverage cans is not a health concern. However, it has been demonstrated that BPA binds to and stimulates the estradiol receptor, tricking the body into thinking estrogen levels are higher than they are. Avoid BPA by choosing fresh over canned foods and avoiding the use of hard plastics.

Like BPA, **phthalates** have been in the news repeatedly. Primarily found in plastics to increase its flexibility, phthalates are not only estrogenic, they have been found to increase programmed cell death (particularly in testicular cells). Phthalates are not bonded to the plastics, and they are fat-soluble—so they therefore leech easily into fatty foods packaged in flexible plastic wrapping. Cosmetics and personal care products also deliver a dose of phthalates topically. Overall, phthalates are linked to breast cancer, birth defects, low sperm count, obesity, diabetes, and thyroid problems. To avoid phthalates, store your food and beverages in glass rather than plastic as much as possible, read labels for personal care items to make sure phthalates are not on the list, make sure you use glass or stainless steel water bottles, and NEVER microwave food with plastic wrap on top! (If you must microwave, use paper towels to avoid splatter instead.)

Polybrominated diphenyl ethers (PBDEs), unfortunately, are just as pervasive as BPA and phthalates. PBDEs are found throughout homes because they are used in fire retardants that are applied to foam furniture, carpets, and a variety of other products. PBDEs also don't break down very well and therefore bioaccumulate. They're everywhere, and they have been shown to decrease fertility and disrupt thyroid activity. Hopefully laws will better protect us in the future and render these less ubiquitous. These can be avoided with very expensive specialty furniture or alternative-type furnishings, but in the meantime, honestly I just don't worry about it. (Can't avoid everything!)

Organophosphate pesticides are equally common. Organophosphate pesticides are some of the most common pesticides in use today, and they are neurotoxic to insects. Unfortunately they're neurotoxic to us as well. For that reason, OP use has been banned in most residential areas, but they're still commonly used on fruits and veggies, and are also used in plastics and as solvents. They've been linked with low testosterone and thyroid disruption. Avoid them by buying the Dirty Dozen fruits and veggies organic, limiting your exposure to solvents, and finding alternatives to plastic.

PFCs, or perfluorinated chemicals, are widely-used endocrine disrupting chemicals. Used in non-stick cookware and water-resistant coatings, these pretty much never break down in the environment.

They have also been linked to low sperm count, kidney and thyroid disease. Instead of the non-stick variety, choose stainless steel pots and pans—I know they're a pain to clean, but they're much safer. Also try to limit your use of disposable tableware and to-go containers.

PFCs are not the only toxin associated with disposable products. **Dioxins** are mostly byproducts of the production of pesticides, waste incineration, and bleaching paper pulp. Unfortunately, they're also tenacious—once they show up in the environment, they're not readily broken down. They hide in fat cells, and most of our exposure actually comes from animals: that is, the animals accumulate them in their fat and then we eat the animal, or drink its milk. Once they're in our bodies, dioxins have half-lives of years. These, too, have endocrine disrupting properties, and have been linked to low sperm count and various kinds of cancer. Avoid these by minimizing agro-industry dairy and meat. Instead, choose organic whenever possible. Also avoid disposable wood pulp products that have extended contact with your skin (think diapers and feminine care products) that do not specifically say that they are dioxin-free.

Atrazine, like dioxin, is another food-contaminating endocrine disrupter. An herbicide used on most corn crops in the US, Atrazine is now a common contaminant in drinking water. Research shows that exposure to even a small amount can turn male frogs into hermaphrodites (with viable eggs!). It is banned in the EU but commonly used in the US and in Australia. Avoid it by choosing organic fruits and veggies, and drinking filtered water (not from a plastic bottle!).

Perchlorate is yet another drinking water contaminant. Referring to a salt with the polyatomic anion perchloric acid, it does occur both naturally and industrially, as it's used in rocket fuel. Because the mineral occurs naturally, it can contaminate drinking water. It inhibits the thyroid's ability to obtain iodine, a necessary mineral for thyroid hormone production, and was therefore once considered the standard of care for hyperthyroidism. However, given today's epidemic of hypothyroidism, it's wise to avoid it and *choose filtered water whenever possible.*

Finally, **glycol ethers** are used as solvents in paint, cleaning solutions, brake fluid, and cosmetics (Did you see that? Cosmetics!). These may lower sperm count, decrease fertility, and they have been associate with allergies and asthma. Avoid them by choosing cleaning products that lack 2-butoxyethanol (EGBE) and methoxydiglycol (DEGME), carefully reading cosmetic labels, and choosing no-VOC paint products.

* * *

Hillary is a 19 year old college student who became ill after first living in a mold-infested house in South America for a semester, and then coming back to the United States and working in a fast food restaurant, where she was exposed to the solvents in industrial cleaning supplies.

She developed Multiple Chemical Sensitivity, breaking out in rashes and hives at the slightest whiff of perfume or fabric softeners among her classmates.

We put Hillary on a full detoxification protocol, involving far infrared sauna, constitutional hydrotherapy, castor oil packs, colonics, as well as a protocol designed to heal her gut. Over the last few months, Hillary's energy and vitality have returned, and her skin has dramatically improved. She still has a long way to go, but she bounces back from unavoidable everyday exposures more quickly than before.

Heavy Metals and Toxic Elements

Heavy metals are getting more and more attention these days as obstacles to cure and even causes of certain illnesses. Here's a quick breakdown of the most common offenders.

Lead. Lead is found in old paint, solder in plumbing (and therefore in drinking water), and even in some herbal remedies imported from overseas. Lead exposure can also be geographical or occupational (living near or working in a lead smelter or lead mine, welding, construction, and manufacture of

232

certain products such as glass, vinyl mini-blinds, and ceramic glaze). Lead initially gets stored in the bones, and is released when bone turnover increases (such as in pregnancy and menopause). It can disrupt the HPA (Hypothalamus-Pituitary-Adrenal) axis, making it harder to deal with stress. In children, lead has been linked with learning and developmental disabilities including lower IQ and ADD. It is also associated with other neurological problems such as depression and anxiety, Alzheimer's, and Parkinson's Disease. It can cause high blood pressure, often poorly or unresponsive to medication. Again, filter your water. (And don't eat your paint, if you live in an old house. Probably don't eat your paint anyway, that's a good rule of thumb.) Also, if you purchase herbal remedies imported from overseas, make sure you do so from a trusted brand that tests for heavy metals and certifies their products are uncontaminated.

Georgia is a menopausal woman I saw during my first year of practice, and she had hypertension unresponsive to most medications—even multiple combinations of medications. In frustration, I finally tested her for heavy metals, having learned as a student that lead gets stored in the bones, and in menopause, when estrogen levels drop and therefore bone begins to break down, lead can release into the bloodstream, causing hypertension. Sure enough, her lead levels were sky high. I referred her for heavy metal chelation therapy to a fellow practitioner I shared an office with at the time. After that, her blood pressure finally became manageable.

You are probably also aware that **mercury** is a relatively common metal that can have toxic effects. Unfortunately, you may not be aware that minuscule mercury exposures are not as safe as you have been told, and may be causing you significant problems. Mercury is found in farmed or Atlantic fish, and also in dental amalgams. If you have a mouth full of mercury fillings, you can let off enough mercury vapor every time you chew that your mouth will exceed OSHA standards for acceptable levels! Mercury used to be used as a preservative in vaccines (called thimerosal), but thimerosal has been eliminated from most vaccines now except for the influenza vaccine. (It is possible to get thimerosal-free flu vaccines, though.)

Mercury concentrates in the nervous system and has been linked to a variety of neurological disorders; it disrupts steroid hormones and potentially interferes with insulin production. It even eats up your body's antioxidant reserves, leaving you vulnerable to oxidative damage. This is probably why it has been linked to an increased risk of cardiovascular disease. Mercury also inhibits your body's ability to make ATP or adenosine triphosphate, the energy currency of the body.

To avoid mercury, choose wild-caught or Pacific

fish, and avoid tuna, orange roughy, swordfish, shark, halibut, and snapper. Consider eating cod, whitefish, tilapia, ocean perch, shrimp, flounder, scallops, clams, and catfish instead. And if you have amalgams and have the money, consider looking into a biological or holistic dentist to replace the fillings.

Aluminum is found in pans for cooking, "tin" foil, aluminum-based antiperspirants, antacids and many other over-the-counter medications, as an adjuvant in vaccines, in processed foods using baking powder (not the same as baking soda,) and self-rising flour (those that don't include yeast). Examples include processed cheese and cheese products, cake mixes, pancake mixes, rising flours, and frozen dough.

Aluminum concentrates in the lungs, bones, and in the nervous system, and there is some evidence that Aluminum may be correlated with the rise in autism.[1] (I am not completely against vaccines, though. More on this in Chapter 12.) Aluminum has also been linked to breast cancer, kidney failure, dementia, Alzheimer's, MS, ALS, and Parkinson's disease.

Be sure to choose non-aluminum based antiperspirants—or just choose a deodorant and not an antiperspirant at all, if you can handle it. Certain natural deodorants work quite well when used in conjunction with a healthy, non-toxic lifestyle. (Remember that sweat is one of the body's mechanisms to eliminate toxins—the more toxic you are, the smellier you tend to be!)

Avoid over-the-counter meds that contain aluminum. Aluminum is sometimes listed as an active and sometimes as an inactive ingredient, so read your labels.

Replace your aluminum pans. Cast iron or stainless steel are a good choice.

Finally, avoid products containing baking powder in the ingredient list, unless specifically stated that it does not contain aluminum. If they don't say that it doesn't, assume that it does. Same goes for self-rising flour.

Arsenic, as mentioned in Chapter 10, is found in non-organic chicken, as well as in seafood, herbicides, and drinking water. Arsenic is a carcinogen, and it also can interfere with the regulation of cortisol, leading to adrenal issues. Be sure to buy your chicken organic, and choose wild-caught, Pacific seafood. And again, filter your water.

Found mostly in cigarettes, **cadmium** also concentrates in the water, air, and soil especially in industrial areas where smelting and refining occurs—thus, it can be found in the food supply in those regions. It is also used in the manufacture of batteries or plastics. Cadmium is a carcinogen that concentrates in the kidneys, liver, and pancreas, but is easily absorbed through the lungs and can can lead to kidney failure, gout, and loss of sense of smell. It is hard to avoid industrial cadmium pollution, but you can certainly stop smoking and limit your exposure to second-hand smoke to avoid much of it.

Fluoride comes from the element fluorine—the most reactive element on the periodic table. Because of this, too much of it can interrupt some of the body's critical activities and act as a poison.

Fluoride concentrates in bones, and because of this, too much fluoride can actually weaken teeth and bones. It has been linked with osteosarcoma, a very aggressive bone cancer. Cosmetically, excessive fluoride can cause enamel fluorosis (mottling or white streaks across the teeth). Fluoride is found in toothpaste and dental care products and is also added to the water supply of many municipalities. You can avoid it by filtering your water and choosing fluoride-free dental products (other toothpastes plus the physical action of brushing will clean your teeth just fine).

But again, you can't avoid everything, and you'd go crazy trying. To minimize the heavy metal exposures that are outside your control, make sure you're getting your daily dose of antioxidants. These will both counter the effects of some heavy metals, and improve your body's natural detoxification mechanisms. Make sure, too, that you're getting your daily dose of chlorophyll. This means eating lots of greens —the darker the better! Also, make sure you're getting your daily dose of fiber. Fiber helps to bind and eliminate toxins of all kinds. Whole grains and veggies are a great source.

Finally, don't forget to drink plenty of water! This flushes out your cells, and helps to prevent constipation, which will impede toxic elimination.

Toxic Skin Products

Skin care and beauty products often contain both the heavy metals and the endocrine disrupting chemicals (aluminum, fluoride, glycol ether) mentioned above. Unfortunately, topical products almost always contain at least some chemicals we don't recognize, even the so-called "clean" ones. That means you've got to read the labels very carefully!

Although many chemical ingredients have an identifiable name, it is worth mentioning that almost every product on the market contains **phthalates**. The phthalates are not listed on the label though— they're hidden under the ingredient, "fragrance." You can bet that if the product is scented with anything other than natural essential oils, it will contain phthalates. For the rare product that is the exception, you can expect them to mention proudly on the label that it is phthalate-free. As mentioned in Chapter 10, phthalates are endocrine disruptors, and are associated with endocrine cancers. They can also damage the liver, kidneys, lungs, and reproductive system. They were banned in the EU in plastic toys, but are still used in plenty of toiletry products.

Phthalates are not the only toxin in your scented products. About 95% of the chemicals used to make fragrances are derived from petroleum or benzene (the latter is very carcinogenic), and many of these are known toxins. They are linked to many allergic reactions and migraine cases, and patients who are chemically sensitive often cannot handle them at all. Fragrances are hard to avoid—they're added to most of the personal care products you purchase. But at least you can avoid them when you have the choice.

One chemically sensitive patient came to see me for the first time just after another patient had left who had worn perfume. I hadn't noticed it, but the chemically sensitive patient told me very pointedly that her last doctor refused service to patients who arrived wearing scented products, and she believed that was a considerate practice. While I never like to offend anyone and I do keep a HEPA filter in my office for that reason, I can see her point—not only do I have plenty of patients who can become ill from expo-

sure to scented products, the scents themselves are unhealthy and should be discouraged.

Sodium Lauryl Sulphate or Sodium Laureth Sulfate (both called **SLS**) are found almost as frequently as phthalates and fragrances. Suspected carcinogens, SLS is linked to kidney and liver damage (and are associated with frequent UTIs), nervous system disruption, eye damage, eczema and dermatitis, and also linked with SLE (Lupus). They have been banned in Europe and Central America.

Only slightly less common that SLS in skin products, **propylene glycol** (found in antifreeze) is found in almost everything—even in many "natural" products, because it is *FDA approved for food use.* Propylene glycol, which has been banned in Europe, is toxic to the nervous system, clogs pores, and can actually speed up skin aging by depleting moisture from deeper skin layers.

Also found in many "natural" products are the **paraben** preservatives. Parabens mimic estrogens and are, unsurprisingly, associated with endocrine (hormonal) cancers. Specifically they have been linked with breast cancer. They are banned in Japan and Sweden, for obvious reasons. The ones you are most likely to encounter are **methylparaben** and **propylparaben**, but avoid any other words with a "paraben" suffix too.

Formaldehyde (aka formalin, formal and methyl aldehyde) is likewise banned in Japan and Sweden, but routinely used in the United States. Formaldehyde is used as a disinfectant and preservative, and it's a suspected carcinogen, especially linked with lung cancer. Exposure in high doses can cause asthma, headaches, eye irritation and upper respiratory irritation (I can attest to this firsthand from anatomy lab in medical school!)

Anything ending in **-ethanolamine (Diethanolamine, Triethanolamine, Monoethanolamine)** should also be avoided. These chemicals are used as emulsifiers and foaming agents. Upon absorption, they become nitrosamines, which can cause cancer. They are also endocrine disruptors and skin irritants.

Toluene is a solvent toxic to the nervous system. It can also damage the liver, cause asthma, and disrupt the endocrine system. It is found mostly in nail-care products, but it is possible to find brands that are toluene-free.

Talc is also rather product specific: it is only found in powder products. Talc increases risk for ovarian cancer specifically, and for urinary tract infections when used in the genital area—so be sure, if you use powder, to choose a powder that is made from cornstarch. Talc is often found in cosmetic powder products, but there does not seem to be a direct link to toxicity from that route of exposure. I would try to avoid it if possible, especially if found in a loose face powder that may be inhaled.

Xylene (aka xytol or dimethylbenzene) is a surfactant (basically a cleanser) often found in cosmetics under the names **Ammonium Xylenesulfonate** and **Sodium Xylenesulfonate**. Xylene can damage your liver, and cause skin and respiratory tract irritation.

Obviously, it can be tough to avoid all of those ingredients. My general rule is, buy products with as few ingredients as possible—and try to stick to those you recognize. (If I just *have* to have a certain type of product, I scan the ingredient list for these primary offenders. If they aren't on there, I go ahead and buy it.)

Does that mean there might still be something on the list that could cause some damage? Yep. But again, we live in a toxic world, and we can't control everything. Do the best you can, and try not to obsess over the rest.

Toxic Cleaning Products

The same companies that make your beauty products tend to make your cleaning products as well.

Cleaning products are regulated even less stringently than toiletries, and usually they have a greater association with acute toxicity. Read your labels, and avoid those that come with a warning, such as "this could be fatal if inhaled," or "contact poison control immediately if X occurs," etc. Others may warn that the product may severely burn eyes and skin, may cause blindness or death (!!), that the vapors are harmful, or that you must use the product only while wearing gloves. Some labels even say things like "contain a substance known in (such-and-such state) to cause cancer," "probably carcinogenic to humans," or "prolonged exposure may cause reproductive and fetal effects." If you read any such warning, avoid!

Also, be wary of cleaning products with vague ingredients. Makers of cleaning products are not required to disclose their ingredients, and so many of them say things like "surfactant" or "solvent," without specifying their chemical nature. Personally this makes me wonder what they've got to hide... particularly because there are so many chemicals that have been linked with diseases, or that have been banned in other countries. I suggest that you avoid these products.

There's a long list of specific ingredients you should try to avoid. But who's going to remember all those names? (Even I have to look them up every time, and I do this for a living.) Again, my rule is, if I don't recognize the name of an ingredient, it doesn't go in my mouth, on my skin, in my hair, or in my house.

There are a number of green cleaning products available, although you should read those labels as well and subject them to the rules above, since some so-called green products are not as harmless as they claim. There are a few household staples that clean just about anything, though, so you shouldn't need to worry about specialty products too much.

A **non-toxic dish soap** will clean just about any surface. (Really, try it.)

If you need scrubbing power or odor elimination (those air fresheners are poisonous!), add **baking soda**. This even works for ovens: Clean your oven by sprinkling baking soda liberally on the bottom. Spray with water, wait 8 hours, and then scrape and wipe the oven clean.

And whatever dish soap and baking soda will not take care of, you can almost guarantee **vinegar** will. Vinegar cuts through grease, sanitizes counter tops (dilute to 50% if you have grout or other acid-sensitive surfaces), cleans windows, and even replaces fabric softener when added to your laundry's rinse cycle.

* * *

Toxins In Our Textiles

Our wardrobes and linen closets contribute to our polluted indoor air, too. Because of the way that our fibers are grown (or created) and the chemical treatments that are put onto the finished products, many of our fabric products are inherently toxic. If that weren't bad enough, the way we care for those items often adds to the chemical burden inside of our homes.

Natural fibers such as cotton, linen, wool, cashmere, silk, and hemp are, in all, a better choice than synthetic fibers. But unfortunately, cotton is one of the top five pesticide-laden crops. Especially for things like pajamas (since you spend so much time in them), it may be worth it to track down organic cotton.

The manufacture of dyes for natural fibers often involves use of heavy metals such as cadmium, cobalt, and antimony. Thankfully, by choosing textiles colored with natural dyes we can avoid yet another source of toxic metals.

Synthetic fabrics, such as acrylic, polyester, acetate, and nylon, are quite flammable, and therefore require additional chemical treatments (such halogenated flame retardants, or HFRs) to meet fire standards. HFRs have been linked to thyroid disruption, reproductive and developmental problems, immune suppression, and cancer.

Both natural and synthetic fabrics are routinely treated to be stain, static, or wrinkle resistant. This means they have added PFCs (perfluorochemicals). Your body cannot eliminate these easily, and they have been linked to reproductive and developmental toxicity, and cancers of the liver and bladder. Thankfully, most products in this category claim this on their tags, so it is not difficult to avoid them.

Aside from what is bonded into the textiles themselves, we release many toxins into our air from our laundering methods. You know now that many detergents have carcinogenic contaminants (unlabelled) and that you can use vinegar to replace those dryer sheets you can smell all the way outside. But perhaps you are not aware that dry cleaning is a common source of solvent exposure. Perchloroethylene, a volatile organic compound (VOC), is the most common dry cleaning agent. It absorbs into the clothing and does not wash out, and can enter the body through the lungs and skin. Long term exposure can cause liver and kidney damage, and causes cancer in animals. If you have items that must have specialty cleaning, eco-friendly dry cleaners use wet-cleaning technology and biodegradable detergents. If you can find one, they're a good alternative. Also, you may consider hand-washing some dry clean only items—often with natural fabrics, dry cleaning is not necessary, or may not be necessary after the first cleaning. The bottom line though, is to avoid dry cleaning... or if you must have it done, hang the clothes in the garage to air out before bringing them inside, and consider wearing undergarments that limit the garment's contact with your skin.

Surprisingly, it is not just the toxins in our clothing that can affect our health, but also the style too. Constrictive fabrics limit lymphatic circulation (essentially recycled blood plasma). Your lymph is necessary for the immune system to remove waste, toxins, pathogens, and cancer cells. If circulation is inadequate, you can end up with fluid buildup in the tissues (edema), and also limit the above necessary functions.

So, be sure to wear clothes that you find comfortable and can move freely in. If you can find them made from untreated natural fibers, so much the better. And give yourself bonus points if they are naturally dyed!

A Word on Smoking

As we have discussed, there are many pollutants that you have the ability to reduce, but there is one that you have more control over: cigarette smoke (and smoke from cigars, pipes, etc.). Aside from the obvious threat of lung cancer, cigarette smoke is associated with a number of other serious diseases, including pancreatic cancer, cardiovascular disease (including strokes, aneurysms, and CHF), COPD, Alzheimer's Disease, and glaucoma—to name a few. It binds irreversibly with hemoglobin and prevents its binding oxygen, leading to hypoxia. Smoke also damages the lining of the blood vessels, thus setting you up for cardiovascular disease, as well as damage to small blood vessels (leading to poor circulation and damage to the eyes and kidneys). This is because cigarette smoke contains a number of chemicals, many of which are carcinogenic. Here's a partial list:

- Benzene, also found in gasoline and a known carcinogen
- Polonium-210, which is radioactive and very toxic
- Vinyl Chloride, also used to make pipes
- Carbon monoxide, also found in car exhaust
- Hydrogen cyanide, used in chemical weapons
- Butane, used in lighter fluid
- Ammonia, used in household cleaners
- Toluene, used in paint thinners
- Cadmium, used in cigarette batteries, a

known carcinogen
- Lead, once used in paint
- Arsenic, used in pesticides.

Okay, so you know you should quit. But how do you go about doing it?

Your PCP may recommend nicotine-containing products that might work for you, such as gum, e-cigarettes, lozenges, patches, nasal sprays, and even a few oral meds that help modulate nicotine cravings. Certainly try this, and if it works for you, great.

If not, one of the most effective treatments I know for smoking cessation is auricular acupuncture. This is especially effective in conjunction with a taper down schedule for cigarettes, replacing them with a botanical or homeopathic combination specifically designed to curb cravings for cigarette smoke. Any withdrawal symptoms should also be minimized with a basic healthy diet: avoid sugar and processed foods, and get some good nutrition.

Also, consider using peer pressure to your advantage. If you publicly announce that you plan to quit, it will (at least for most people) motivate you to stick with it—if the horrific list of possible smoking-affiliated ailments isn't enough!

Ways to Detox the Air in Your House

Indoor air is typically two to five times more polluted than outdoor air. This is due to things like Volatile Organic Compounds (VOCs) from paint, furniture and flooring, as well as various toxic compounds in cleaning products, self-care products, dry cleaning products… you get the idea.

After tackling heavy metals, non-stick dishes, cleaning products, personal care products, textiles, and (if it applied to you) quitting smoking, your air should feel much fresher. Now that we have removed many of the air polluters, there are some extra steps we can take to really clean up what remains. Just a few simple changes can dramatically improve the quality of the air in your home.

The easiest thing to do is to open a window (or two, or three.) This will at least dilute the polluted indoor air. If you need more air coming into your house, place a fan in front of the window, facing inside. If you are using something toxic, do the opposite and point the fan outside. Because the bathroom air is even more polluted than the rest of the house, your bathroom should have an exhaust fan, and you should use it. If your bathroom has a window, so much the better—and you should definitely be running the fan and/or opening a window if you must use toxic cleaning products! The same goes for your kitchen: if you have a vented range hood, use it. Bedrooms, on the other hand, don't have ventilation fans, but because you spend about a third of your life in your bedroom you want to make sure it has really clean air. Consider getting an air filter for your bedroom; High-Efficiency Particulate Air (HEPA) filters should be able to filter air up to 15 times per hour, and there are also air purifiers with carbon filters available if you still have a source of VOCs. At the very least, if you must use cleaning products containing undisclosed or harmful chemicals for some reason, make sure you open a window, use a fan, or both.

Detoxing Your Body

We have discussed limiting your exposure to known toxins as much as you can by choosing your cleaning products, toiletry items, and food with care, but no matter how hard you try, you won't be able to avoid all toxic exposure. To keep toxic burden low on a regular basis, try incorporating some detox rituals into your daily or weekly routine.

An easy detoxification method to incorporate into your routine is dry brushing your skin before you shower. Even though it seems like this isn't doing much, dry skin brushing (from outer limbs towards the body's core) follows the line of lymphatic drainage. As mentioned above, your lymph is sort of a sewage system for toxins carried by your blood. Dry skin brushing helps to move toxins along so that they can reach some of the key elimination organs to be eliminated.

One patient I saw recently had edema (extra fluid in her lower legs), and for the life of us, we couldn't figure out the cause. I tested her for hypothyroidism, for kidney problems, for cardiac issues, for hormone imbalance problems, and for food allergies—but it wasn't until she started getting lymphatic massage that the edema went away! The implication here was that the valves in her blood vessels weren't as efficient at pushing blood back to the heart as they should have been, allowing blood to stagnate and lymph to pool. Lymphatic massage took care of the problem!

On the days that you are not dry brushing before your shower, make sure you sweat. Get up and get moving! Many toxins are fat-soluble, and sweat helps liberate them from the fat cells and usher them into the bloodstream, where they will eventually find their way to the liver, and, if all works well, into the gut and out of the body.

You can support your liver in removing those toxins by eating more cruciferous veggies. Cruciferous veggies are the ones that "flower outward"—like broccoli, cauliflower, bok choy, and brussels sprouts.

These are excellent support for the liver detoxification pathways.

Eating plenty of fermented foods supports the next stop in the toxin removal pathway: your gut. Fermented foods are packed with probiotics, which are extremely important for your digestive health. An integral part of the raw diet, these used to be a much bigger component of our diets than they are today.

If you want to liberate even more stored toxins, try juicing your veggies. I don't always recommend juicing over eating the veggies whole, particularly if you have insulin resistance, candida overgrowth, or sugar addiction, because juicing removes the fiber and leaves the sugar. But it also leaves the nutrients, and does not require much effort on the part of your digestive system in order to absorb them: perfect for cleansing purposes.

Summary:

- Read labels, not only on your food, but also on your cleaning products and personal care products. If you don't recognize the ingredients (or worse, if they're on the known avoid list), don't buy it.
- Filter your water, and drink plenty of it!
- Buy your fish wild caught, and Pacific or

Alaskan, not Atlantic.
- Stop smoking
- Open your windows!
- If you have a fan or a filter in your kitchen or bathroom, use it as often as possible.
- Either don't dry-clean, or use organic or 'green' dry cleaning instead.
- Consider getting organic cotton pajamas, and avoid synthetic materials.
- Choose cast iron or stainless steel for cooking
- Exercise!

CHAPTER 12

Chapter 12: Obstacle to Cure #3: Toxic Buildup from Pharmaceuticals

Before I launch into the down side of pharmaceuticals, let me just state that I am not against them. I do prescribe medications, and I'm very grateful to have a scope of practice that allows me to do this. I just don't prescribe them *first*, not usually.

For a little perspective: infectious disease was the number one killer in 1900, accounting for 32 percent of all deaths. Mortality declined even prior to the invention of penicillin in 1935 due to improved nutrition and public health measures, but it dropped twice as fast in the period between 1940 and 1960, when antibiotics were added to the mix. This trend leveled off after 1960, and our mortality rates now, though still declining, are declining at roughly the same rate as they were in the pre-antibiotics era. (Now we're dying for other reasons—namely heart disease and cancer.)

Antibiotics: Good or Bad?

The "germ theory of disease" was essentially the work of Louis Pasteur (hence the word *pasteurization*, a process that uses high heat to kill off bacteria)—he's the guy who said that each type of bacteria caused a specific kind of illness.

Nobody ever hears about Pasteur's contemporary, though—he was a guy named Antoine Bechamp, who said essentially the opposite. Bechamp claimed that there was a symbiotic relationship between bacteria and their hosts, and that bacteria can morph to adopt to their environments. In other words, when you try to kill a certain type of bacteria, most of them might die, but *the few that remain will pass on their resistance to their progeny.*

Turns out they were both right. Pasteur was correct in that there are some organisms so pathogenic that your immune system isn't likely to be able to overcome them without some outside intervention, no matter how strong you may be. There are also some individuals whose immune function is so weakened that they won't be able to overcome an infectious invader without outside intervention, even if the invader itself isn't all that strong. These are situations in which antibiotics are absolutely appropriate.

However, Bechamp's discoveries should not be overlooked either. Antibiotics are usually indiscriminate, which means they kill not just the bacteria causing symptoms, but they also slaughter all of the "good," symbiotic bacteria in our guts (aka probiotics, as discussed in Chapter 3), which contribute substantially to the health of our immune system, thus rendering us far more susceptible to future invaders. Then, when those future invaders arrive, instead of strengthening the immune system to fight them off naturally, we throw another round of antibiotics at them, weakening the system still further.

Additionally, this approach allows those previously symbiotic organisms that survive in the gut to overgrow and create imbalance. Certain bacteria and yeast that are helpful in small amounts can create gas, bloating, constipation, food allergies, brain fog and a number of other symptoms when they are allowed to overpopulate in order to fill the void that the antibiotics left behind (see Chapter 14).

Overexposure to antibacterial products can also contribute to weakened immune function such as allergies and increased susceptibility to pathogens. Even worse, triclosan, the antibiotic most frequently used in antibacterial household products such as soap, can form toxic byproducts when combined with the chlorine in water, such as carcinogenic dioxins, and has been linked with disrupted thyroid function.

Ultimately my conclusion on antibiotics is very much the way I view pharmaceuticals generally: they are powerful tools, to be used in appropriate conditions (such as those Pasteur identified). But overuse will cause us to fall into the trap Bechamp outlined: imbalance, weakened immune function, resistant bacteria, and increased susceptibility.

Vaccines: the Pros and Cons

Both antibiotics and vaccines have undoubtedly saved many lives. There was a time when there was absolutely no question that the risks of not vaccinating were much higher than the risks of choosing to vaccinate. Yet now, Pediatrician Dr Lawrence Palevsky says in the documentary, *The Greater Good*[1]: "The science is not there to really state that vaccines are truly safe." Specifically, there are no studies to determine whether vaccine quantities of additives and adjuvants, such as aluminum and thimerosol (mercury), are safe long-term. In larger quantities, aluminum and mercury are both neurotoxic (see Chapter 11)—that is not in question.

The conventional medical community argues that there are in fact six studies that state that vaccines are not connected with autism, though, and therefore are safe.

According to The National Vaccine Information Center's Barbara Fisher, the placebos in vaccine trials have the same questionable adjuvants in them as the vaccines themselves, and are therefore not true placebo trials.[1]

On the other side of the argument, there's the concept of herd immunity. The idea is that if enough people in a given population are immunized against a particular illness, an outbreak cannot occur—thus protecting those who are too young or weak or immunocompromised to receive vaccines.

I see quite a few patients with Multiple Chemical Sensitivity (MCS) in my practice, most of whom have family members who have suffered the exact same exposures and are not similarly ill. All people cannot detoxify equally, that much is evident; so it stands to reason that not all kids can tolerate the same burden from vaccine adjuvants equally. If that's the case, how much damage are we doing with the mandated vaccine schedule, irrespective of the individual child?

What Can We Do About It?

Ultimately in my view, the question of vaccination comes down to a cost/benefit analysis. First, look at each individual vaccine, and compare the risks associated with that particular vaccine with the risks of the disease, should your child contract it, and the likelihood of your child's exposure to the illness. Some vaccines confer higher risks, and protect against an illness to which it is quite unlikely your child will be exposed. But others are relatively low risk, and protect against potentially fatal illnesses, to which your child could conceivably be exposed. *The Vaccine Book* by Dr Robert Sears does a great job of outlining the pros and cons, but here's a cursory overview of what I believe to be the salient points.

- **Hep B (Hepatitis B):** this vaccine is given immediately after birth (with two more boosters later), and it is necessary if mom has Hep B, because then the baby will be exposed. Otherwise, it is transferred almost exclusively via sexual or blood contact, and children are therefore unlikely to be exposed until adolescence. It's unclear whether immunity will last into adulthood.
- **RV (Rotavirus)**: this is a bigger issue in third world countries than in the US. Less than ten kids in the US die of Rotavirus yearly; if they catch it they'll typically get symptoms such as a runny nose, fever,

or at worst, watery diarrhea (which can cause dehydration—and this could be concerning depending on the size and age of the child).

- **DTaP (Diphtheria, Tetanus, Pertussis)**: usually a series of five shots, although it can be four depending on the age of the child.

  - *Diphtheria* is basically obsolete in the US but it's part of the series, so you don't really get to pick on this one—it's all or nothing.

  - *Tetanus:* once kids start walking, they may run the risk of, for instance, stepping on a rusty nail and contracting this. It's a serious and rapidly fatal infection, and although you can just get the tetanus shot after exposure, by the time you realize you've been exposed it's already too late.

  - *Pertussis*: if a baby contracts this under three months of age, it's rapidly fatal. Older people, however, only get an annoying and persistent cough. The most common route of transmission to a newborn is through a family member, so it's often recommended for the adults in the newborn's household.

- **Hib (Haemophilus Influenzae)**: This is a four dose series typically. Infection can lead to epiglottitis (which closes the throat) and meningitis (infection of the tissue surrounding the brain), both of which are serious and potentially fatal. On the other hand, the vaccine itself has been associated with autoimmune disease.

- **PCV (Pneumococcal Conjugate Vaccine)**: this is usually a four dose series vaccine against the most common strains of streptococcus pneumoniae, which (hence the name) can cause pneumonia, but can also cause meningitis in infants, and this can be very serious or fatal. However, the vaccine is live, which can make it tougher for a little one to handle if given in conjunction with other live vaccines.
- **IPV (Inactivated Polio Vaccine)**: Polio is still common in India and Africa... not so much in the US. However, polio can have debilitating and lasting effects.
- **Influenza**: this is also a live vaccine, which means you can get the flu from the vaccine itself. It's very rare for a child to die of the flu if he or she does get it. At the time of this writing, some flu vaccines still have thimerosol (mercury) in them but some do not—you can request those that don't.
- **MMR (Measles Mumps Rubella)**: this vaccine contains three live viruses at once, which can overwhelm an immature immune system. This is also the vaccine most frequently connected with autism, though the debate on this point is quite heated. It has also been associated with ITP (Idiopathic Thromobocytopenia Purpura), or low platelets that lead to bruising with no clear cause.

- *Rubella:* if babies get this it isn't a very big deal, but if a pregnant woman catches it, it can harm the fetus.

- *Mumps*: this can cause meningitis, but it is not as virulent as the form conferred by H. flu (Hib) or strep pneumo (PCV). It also has been linked to orchitis and sterility in teenage boys. But protection from childhood vaccination does not last into adulthood, so the traditional vaccine schedule includes a booster around 4-6 years.

- *Measles:* it's miserable—the kid gets a high fever, a rash, lots of upper respiratory symptoms, and it's quite contagious... but, all else being equal, they'll fight it off and be fine. It can cause meningitis and encephalitis (inflammation of the brain itself,) but it usually doesn't.

- **Varicella (chicken pox)**: this is also a live vaccine. Kids can die from chicken pox, although they usually don't. There is a chance that chicken pox sores can get infected and cause scarring, though. Older kids who catch the chicken pox have a much more severe case than younger kids, and if a pregnant woman gets it, it can cause deafness in the fetus. There is an increased rate of shingles post-vaccination, even in kids.

- **MCV (Meningococcal Vaccines)**: this form of meningitis is particularly nasty, and once you

catch it, it's hard to treat—about 50% of those infected die from it, although death tends to occur around
16-20 years of age. For this reason, first vaccination
is recommended at around 11 years, with a booster
several years later to ensure continued protection.
Some neurological side effects (Guillain Barre syndrome) are associated with the vaccine, although
rarely.

When deciding on a particular vaccine, I'd add to
this one more question: has the child ever had an adverse vaccine reaction in the past, or is there any reason to suspect that he or she does not detoxify well?
Genetic testing has been very helpful in confirming
what I've already suspected in my chemically sensitive patients: every time, the liver cytochrome systems have multiple heterozygous, if not homozygous
mutations, rendering detoxification more
challenging.

Next, I'd look at the overall vaccine schedule,
which is fortunately only recommended in the state
of AZ, but is mandated in many other states. In the
1980s children were asked to get 23 doses of 7 vaccines. At the time, autism occurred in 1 out of every
10,000 children[3]. In the last 3 decades, the schedule
has grown to 69 doses of 16 vaccines, or three times
as many vaccines at once. Now, autism has swelled

to 1 in 50^4, and rates continue to increase by 10-17% per year. During that same period of time, we've also seen an explosion in chronic disease, developmental delays, and disabilities in children. One in six children in this country has some form of neurodevelopment disability.

Correlation is not causation, of course. Vaccinations are not the only thing that have changed in our environment since the 1980s. Undoubtedly we live in a toxic soup, and vaccine preservatives and adjuvants are only one part of that. I've certainly heard mothers of autistic children say that their children were neurotypical until vaccination, at which point everything changed... but those are anecdotal stories, not true scientific studies.

We need the studies. We need objective data, comparing vaccinations with true placebos on a wide enough scale that the data will mean something. Until then, at the very least I believe that the vaccination schedule ought to be modified.

Other Pharmaceuticals: Benzodiazepines and Antidepressants

Benzodiazepines and antidepressants are particularly troubling because, while there are people who truly benefit from them, they are often prescribed to people that do not need psychiatric help. Rather, they need medical help that consists of a proper diagnosis and treatment, and an acknowledgment that many mood problems are actually a side effect of a *physical* ailment. In these circumstances, Selective Serotonin Reuptake Inhibitors (SSRIs) and their brethren are used to mask symptoms by altering biochemistry, and this is not a good thing.

We tend to think of antidepressants and anti-anxiety meds (benzodiazepines) as "silver bullets," much in the same way that we originally viewed antibiotics in the days of Louis Pasteur. The idea that depression and anxiety are caused by chemical imbalance in the brain is so widespread that it almost goes without question… and antidepressants especially (and benzodiazepines as well) supposedly correct those chemical imbalances, helping such afflicted individuals function normally in society.

But there isn't any evidence for that hypothesis.

The theory of depression as a chemical imbalance in the brain was first postulated by Bernard Brodie.[5] But when depressed patients and normal controls were tested for the breakdown products of serotonin (5-HIAA), researchers failed to find a statistically significant difference between the two—nor did there appear to be any correlation between 5-HIAA levels and depressive symptoms.[6,7] Further studies showed that depressed patients who had not taken antidepressants had normal 5-HIAA levels.[8]

Stanford psychiatrist David Burns said in 2003, "I spent the first several years of my career doing full-time research on brain serotonin metabolism, but I never saw any convincing evidence that any psychiatric disorder, including depression, results from a deficiency of brain serotonin."[9]

Colin Ross, associate psychiatry professor of Southwest Medical Center in Dallas, said, "There is no scientific evidence whatsoever that clinical depression is due to any kind of biological deficit state."[10]

Depressed patients treated with SSRIs end up with a chemical imbalance as a result of the drugs, though.

Your body is a living system, designed to find balance (homeostasis) with its environment. SSRIs (Selective Serotonin Reuptake Inhibitors) prevent serotonin from being recycled, so it sticks around to re-stimulate its receptors longer. Your brain responds to this by decreasing the number of serotonin receptors it produces, because it thinks you have too much serotonin already. So your body drops the production of serotonin receptors by 25% within four weeks,[11] and up to 50% with chronic use.[12] This may also be the reason why it takes 3-4 weeks for SSRIs to "work."

Antipsychotics do essentially the same thing with the dopamine system instead of serotonin, but instead they block the dopamine receptors, forcing the body to flood the system with more and more dopamine.

Benzodiazepines increase the affinity of receptors for the calming neurotransmitter GABA. This leads to a decrease in the inhibitory effects of GABA, as well as an increase in the excitatory neurotransmitter glutamate to compensate.

In other words, you may not have had a chemical imbalance before, but you will after taking these drugs. That's why you can't abruptly stop any of the psych drugs without potentially severe consequences.

The introduction of these drugs to the public has also corresponded with a dramatic decline in American mental health.

In 1955, only one in every 468 Americans was considered to be mentally disabled, and there were only 5,415 "psychoneurotic" (anxiety disorder) patients in state mental hospitals.[13]

Then Valium (a benzodiazepine) hit the market in 1963. It was the bestselling drug in the Western world until 1981, touted as perfectly safe. It works very quickly to calm anxiety, but the clinical trials demonstrate (and most people can attest) that these benefits are pretty much gone by 4-6 weeks.[14] But the withdrawal symptoms were so horrific and in many cases so lingering[15] that in 1975, the U.S. Justice Department made it a controlled substance (schedule IV drug). Patients who remain on benzos long-term have a four-fold increase in depressive symptoms, as well as a gradual increase in panic attacks and agoraphobia.[16] The "higher the intake, dose and period of use [of benzodiazepines], the greater the risk of impairment."[17]

By 2006 more than 300,000 adults in the US were on SSI (government disability) for anxiety disorder alone—that's about 60 times the number hospitalized for psychoneurosis (anxiety) in 1955.[18]

In the 1930s and 1940s, less than one in a thousand adults suffered clinical depression yearly.[13] Around 60 percent of such individuals suffered only a single episode of depression in their lifetimes, and only 13 percent suffered three or more episodes.[19] Dean Schuyler, head of the depression section at the NIMH in 1974, noted that spontaneous recovery rates for depression exceeded 50 percent within a few months.[20]

Then Prozac was approved in 1987. While depression had previously been associated with a high rate of spontaneous recovery within a few months to a year and a low relapse rate, studies show that the longer the duration of treatment with SSRIs, the higher the rate of relapse.[21] In fact, those treated for depression were three times more likely than untreated depressed patients to "suffer a cessation of their principle social role, and nearly seven times more likely to become incapacitated."[22]

All told, in 2007 the disability rate had soared to one in every 76 Americans, from one in every 468 Americans in 1955.[23] This includes children—in 1987, pre-Prozac, only 5.5 percent of American kids were on disability rolls for mental health issues. By 2007 that number rose thirty five fold, and is now the leading cause of disability in children.[24] By June 2008, one in every sixteen young adults is now considered to be mentally ill.[25]

Once again, correlation is not causation. But the statistics, along with what I know of the body's homeostatic mechanisms and the implications of how that might apply to psych meds, are enough to concern me.

If that weren't enough, consider the common side

effects of Prozac (an SSRI): nausea, headache, insomnia, nervousness, anxiety, asthenia (weakness), diarrhea, anorexia, dizziness, xerostomia (dry mouth), tremor, dyspepsia (indigestion), diaphoresis (unusual sweating), ejaculatory dysfunction, constipation, decreased libido, rash, visual disturbance, and urinary disorders.

Kelli came to me a few months after the birth of her third child, having suffered from postpartum depression. Her PCP put her on an SSRI, and while she said the drug took the edge off of her depression, she was still depressed—and worse, now she also had no libido, headaches, a flat affect, and no energy. We tapered her off the drug, gave her a homeopathic medication specific to hormonal depression, supported her adrenals, and discussed ways to rearrange her schedule such that she was sleeping more and prioritizing only necessary activities. She now reports that she is back to her old self, her libido is back, headaches are gone, and with a few adjustments in her commitments, her energy also improved.

And that's not all! The serious side effects are depression exacerbation and/or suicidality (ironic, no?), mania, serotonin syndrome (a possibly fatal overload of serotonin in the central nervous system), extrapyramidal symptoms (involuntary movement), hyponatremia (low sodium), inappropriate water excretion, seizures, hypoglycemia, anaphylactoid reactions, serum sickness, vasculitis, severe skin rashes and hypersensitivity conditions, pulmonary fibrosis, disruptions of the heart's electrical cycle and resultant tachycardia, abnormal bleeding and/or abnormal platelet function, glaucoma, priapism (penile erection lasting more than four hours), and hypotension.

There are also withdrawal symptoms if the drugs are stopped abruptly. In addition, pediatric patients may have suppressed growth. Finally, if used during the third trimester of pregnancy, the infant could have withdrawal symptoms or neonatal serotonin syndrome after delivery.

The common side effects of Xanax (a benzodiazepine for anxiety) are: drowsiness, fatigue, impaired coordination, irritability, amnesia, appetite changes, confusion, dysarthria (inarticulate speech), dizziness, impaired concentration, xerostomia, libido changes, urinary retention, menstrual irregularities, sialorrhea (drooling), hypotension, rash, diplopia (double vision), high liver enzymes, disinhibition, and incontinence.

Xanax, too, has a number of serious side effects: dependency and/or abuse of the medication, respiratory depression, seizures, suicidality, tachycardia, severe hypotension, paradoxical central nervous system stimulation, liver toxicity, Stevens-Johnson syndrome (a life-threatening skin condition), angioedema, and, of course, withdrawal symptoms if stopped abruptly.

While many of my patients have successfully tapered off benzodiazepines without incident, I vividly remember June. She was 38 years old and came to me with the most severe speech disturbance I had ever encountered—it took her quite a long while to articulate each sentence, and the visit progressed slowly. She also had spasmodic tics, mostly jerking her head to her shoulder. Had I seen her on the street, I would likely have assumed she was on recreational drugs, but in fact her symptoms were a result of prolonged benzodiazepine usage. She had tried many times to get off but could not seem to slow down enough to avoid serious withdrawals. Unfortunately I was unable to help her, because she did not trust any recommendations I made, even homeopathics or supplements. She had been so badly harmed by recommendations from doctors in the past that by the time I saw her, she was unwilling even to make dietary adjustments.

Of course, psychiatric drugs are not the only medications that are prescribed unnecessarily, nor are they the only prescriptions with a long list of damaging side effects. An estimated 32 million Americans are on statins, due to our obsession with lowering cholesterol (which you now know is not the real enemy, as mentioned in Chapter 1).

Statins

Fat and cholesterol are necessary for the formation and maintenance of healthy cellular membranes (including those of neurons, enabling easy transmission and uptake of neurotransmitters), the formation of all cholesterol-based hormones and neurotransmitters, and the maintenance of healthy mucous membranes. Not surprisingly, patients on statin drugs to lower their cholesterol must monitor their other cholesterol-based hormones carefully, and are likely to experience a wide variety of side effects.

The common side effects for Simvastatin, for example, are abdominal pain, constipation, upper respiratory symptoms, flatulence, diarrhea, asthenia, diabetes mellitus, myalgia (muscle pain), elevated CK levels (usually indicators of muscle or heart damage), elevated liver enzymes, and cognitive impairment. The more serious side effects of Simvastatin are immune-mediated myopathy (muscular disease), rhabdomyolysis (a potentially fatal breakdown of skeletal muscle), acute renal failure, liver toxicity, pancreatitis, hypersensitivity reactions such as erythema multiforme, anaphylaxis, photosensitivity, Stevens-Johnson syndrome, toxic epidermal necrolysis, thrombocytopenia (platelet deficiency), and leukopenia (a reduction in white blood cells).

When I need to lower a patient's cholesterol, my first choice is of course to modify diet. I also may throw in either lecithin or inositol hexaniacinate, both

supplements, or perhaps cholestyramine, a medication I usually prescribe for mold exposure but which
was originally designed to bind and eliminate cholesterol from the body. Red Yeast Rice also works well,
because it does contain a botanical statin (without
anywhere near the side effect profile of the drug version). I always make sure I'm combining these treatments with a diet and lifestyle intervention to treat
the root cause, of course.

Contraceptive Side Effects

Like statins, birth control medications are also a
very popular type of prescription drug. Many doctors
will prescribe hormone-based birth control pills in an
effort to regulate a woman's cycle. These are often
effective, and while many women do fine on them,
there are some long-term consequences which you
should keep in mind, such as increased risk of certain
cancers and of stroke (especially for women over 35
who smoke).

One popular hormonal contraceptive pill is Yasmin. Its side effects have spurred lawsuits, but it is
still regularly prescribed. Yasmin's side effects include breast pain or tenderness, headaches, non-men-
strual vaginal bleeding, irregular menstrual periods,
nausea and/or vomiting, longer and/or heavier men-

strual periods, general tiredness or weakness, chills, candidiasis (yeast infections), urinary tract infections, upper respiratory infections, difficulty breathing, dizziness, fever, itching, loss of appetite or increased appetite, pain in the chest, groin, or legs, rash, slurred speech, sudden loss of coordination, sudden severe limb weakness, halitosis, vision changes, vomiting of blood, crying, decreased libido, delusions and/or combativeness, irritability, depression, emotional overreaction, mood swings, weight gain, acne, hair loss, hypertension, increased serum potassium levels, jaundice, amenorrhea, melasma, edema, exacerbations of Lupus, porphyria, and chorea, diminished lactation, flu syndrome, tooth disorder, infection, aggravation of varicose veins, heart attack, stroke, vascular thrombosis (blood clots) or embolism, changes in plasma lipid profiles and carbohydrate metabolism, lowered glucose tolerance levels, gallbladder disease, esophageal ulceration, retinal thrombosis, optic neuritis, osteonecrosis (bone death), and benign migratory glossitis. There are also, as mentioned previously, associations with breast cancer, cervical cancer, and liver cancer.[22] Most other hormonal birth control options contain a side effect profile that includes at least some of those problems on this list.

My recommendations for birth control depend on

the couple, their values and goals. My current favorite, which I was not taught about in medical
school but had to learn about later, is the Fertility
Awareness Method. This is not the same as the
Rhythm Method, which is notoriously ineffective and
relies on the (often false) assumption that a woman
ovulates on Day 14 of her cycle. The Fertility Awareness Method involves charting both the woman's cervical fluid throughout her cycle and her temperatures.
While it takes more effort at first, and works best
with monogamous couples and with abstinence during the woman's fertile period (or at least with two
barrier methods and spermicide during that time), it
is the only truly natural birth control method I know
of and avoids all the drawbacks of hormonal
methods, the heavy periods and cramping of IUDs,
and the inconvenience of barriers all cycle long. For
more on this, I recommend the definitive textbook on
the subject, *Taking Charge of Your Fertility,* by Toni
Weschler.[27]

It *is* possible to use prescription medication without having any of the listed side effects, of course.
But even if you manage to escape those, they will
likely leave a toxic burden for your body to deal
with. Usually, the stress from this is focused on your
liver, which is one of your body's main cleansing organs.

* * *

Identifying a Toxic Liver

Think of your liver like your body's trash bucket. When you're born, it's empty (or at least it is for most of us). As you go through life, you encounter toxins, chemicals, organisms, and complex molecules that your body has to break down in order for them to be eliminated. These molecules get funneled into your "trash bucket"… and as long as it can keep up with the demand, you're okay. But as soon as the trash bucket gets too full, suddenly anything you try to throw into it spills out onto the floor (which in this case is your bloodstream). After that, even the most minor encounter with a substance that your liver would ordinarily need to process in order for elimination to occur will lead to symptoms. There are five typical ways that this presents: chemical sensitivity, allergies, hormonal problems, mold sensitivity, and mental health issues.

You know your liver needs cleansing if you're really sensitive to chemicals. Patients with chemical sensitivities often say they have a major aversion to perfume, or cigarette smoke. Often they may have lived in a house under new construction (new materials tend to off-gas a lot), or worked in a building known to be toxic. Some will say they cannot handle using normal cleaning supplies, or even walking down the cleaning aisle at the store. Some have a hard time in big box stores (often cheaper clothing contains traces of formaldehyde). Some even swell up and develop itchy eyes or skin in the shower, as a reaction to the chlorine in tap water.

In addition to chemical sensitivity, it is pretty standard for liver toxicity to result in out-of-control allergies. Allergens are substances that are not inherently harmful to the body, but the body reacts as if they were harmful—the same way it might react to a pathogen. If the liver gets overwhelmed with toxins, either because of a massive exposure or because of cumulative exposures, it will store those excess toxins until it can get to them and produce histamine (signaling invasion to the body). This is the reason why we suddenly develop seasonal allergies when the concentration of pollen in the air spikes, and the reason why some of us, as we get more "toxic," struggle with allergies all year round. Note that high tendency towards allergies, especially food allergies, almost guarantees adrenal fatigue as well as liver toxicity (more on this in Chapter 16).

Our livers don't just filter toxins, they are also responsible for breaking down and eliminating our hormones. If your hormones are out of whack, it may be a signal that your liver is too busy detoxing chemicals or dealing with allergens. When chemicals and allergens get backed up, hormones get backed up too. This leads to recycling sex hormones, which can severely exacerbate or even cause PMS and menopausal symptoms (see Chapter 17).

Sensitivity to mold is both a cause of liver toxicity *and* a clue that the liver is toxic. Some molds produce mycotoxins (mold toxins) that are extremely poisonous to the body. This exposure typically happens through environmental exposure (most often in water damaged homes or buildings) or though food contamination. Because of the mycotoxins, some mold exposure can really clog up the liver, leading to all of these symptoms. I often see cases of inexplicable chemical sensitivities, allergies, and a host of physical symptoms all beginning with acute or severe exposure to mold.

Andrea came to me with IBD (Crohn's Disease), severe constipation, nausea, and tremors—all starting when she and her family moved into a moldy house. She was no longer in that house by the time I saw her, but she could make no headway with the rest of her condition. We put her on cholestyramine to help remove mold from her body, as well as homeopathic Ipecac for nausea, absorbable magnesium as a non-habit forming laxative to bowel tolerance, and the Specific Carbohydrate Diet along with glutamine and probiotics to help heal up her gut lining. Several months later, Andrea reported a return of energy, normal bowel movements and food tolerance for the first time in years.

Sometimes, in addition to physical symptoms, there can be mental health clues as well. If you are emotionally unbalanced, it may be a sign of liver toxicity. It can also be a lot of other things, of course. From a Chinese Medicine standpoint, though, the liver regulates and governs emotions. I will also say that low adrenal function is often also a culprit for uncharacteristic emotional instability (see Chapter 16).

If any of the above describes you, it is a sign that your liver may need some attention and a little assistance in doing its job.

Liver Cleansing Approaches

I tend to favor nutritional and (sometimes) mechanical approaches to liver cleansing over supplementation alone, as I often do not think supplements alone are strong enough to effect the quick change I'd like to see. Nutritional approaches include fasting in various forms, including water and juice fasts or guided medical food fasts. I use fasting as a sort of "reset button," decreasing overall inflammation in the body and allowing the liver and GI to flush out toxins. When the cleanse or fast is over, a clearer picture emerges of what still needs to be treated. If you fast, make sure you drink LOTS of water! This also helps your body to flush out toxins, much like rinsing out a bucket helps it get clean.

Mechanical approaches to detox include infrared sauna, hydrotherapy, castor oil packs, and enemas or colon hydrotherapy. This approach helps your body physically remove toxins from the fat cells (where many of them are stored if they don't make it all the way to the liver), and helps flush them out of your body.

If you've been acutely exposed to mold, however, you will probably require pharmaceutical treatment (cholestyramine or colestipol) for complete elimination. And, in this case, the relatively benign side effects are much better than the long-term damage done by carrying a burden of mycotoxins in your body!

Summary:

Pharmaceuticals have their place in acute care. However, over time prescription or over the counter meds can cause toxic buildup that can become an obstacle to cure. The same rules apply: minimize exposure as much as you can, taper off of medications that cannot be abruptly stopped, and give your liver as much love and support as you can!

Chapter 13

Obstacle to Cure #4: Toxic Buildup from Stress

Chemicals and other toxins are certainly important, but I would be remiss if I did not discuss the topic of stress. Stress is *the* most pervasive toxin we have. None of us is immune.

How Stress Affects Your Mind

For many of us, our minds show symptoms of stress before our bodies. Here's what it looks like (in one variety).

The common culture of the American workplace, filled with myriad distractions, high pressure, noise, and multitasking leads us to an environmental product called *Attention Deficit Trait (ADT)*. People working with ADT find it difficult to prioritize, stay organized, and manage time effectively. This leads to a downward spiral of decreasing productivity, and increasing angst. Very commonly patients with apparent ADT tell me that they "can't shut off their brains," especially at night—they lie awake for hours, or wake in the wee hours of the morning, trying to solve the problems that confront them during the day. They tend to be anxious and irritable, and while some take this irritability out on their coworkers or loved ones, others will turn it inward, blaming themselves.

Think of these symptoms as early warning signals. If the problem is your environment, medicating yourself so that you can better cope with it is sort of like turning off the fire alarm when your house is on fire, instead of grabbing the extinguisher. Eventually the house is still going to burn down, whether you sleep through it or not.

If you choose to ignore the warning symptoms, your stress will continue to grow and will eventually start impacting you physically.

How Stress Affects Your Body

Your adrenals are these two pyramid-shaped glands that sit on top of your kidneys. They've got several jobs, but the biggest is to help your body cope with stress.

If you were to get attacked by a bear, without sparing the critical seconds necessary to talk to your Central Nervous System (CNS), the core of your adrenals would flood your body with adrenaline directly—it's an automatic response. This makes your heart race, your bronchioles dilate, and provides your muscles with immediate blood flow (oxygen and glucose for energy) to get away quickly or fight, if it comes to that. The adrenaline also overrides this little "gatekeeper" in your muscles called the golgi tendon organ. The job of the golgi tendon organ is to prevent over-strain on the muscles. If you're fighting for your life, that's not important, though—and this is the reason why a flood of adrenaline can allow people to perform superhuman feats, like a mother lifting a car off of her baby.

After you've either killed or gotten away from the bear, the outside of your adrenals produces another hormone called cortisol. Due to the rush of adrenaline, you've just consumed massive sugar reserves (so now you're probably shaky and hypoglycemic), your blood pressure and heart rate are really high, and your body has totally neglected normal life maintenance stuff like digesting your food and repairing your tissues. Cortisol helps to restore this balance. It encourages the breakdown of glycogen (stored glucose) and gluconeogenesis (production of new glucose from fat in the liver). It redirects blood flow to repair tissues and digest food. It's basically the natural steroid of your body (the equivalent of prednisone, though not nearly as strong), so it's an anti-inflammatory as well… and also an immune suppressant. (This is because you shouldn't spare the energy to fight off a cold when you're busy running from a bear. Survival takes precedence.)

This system is only designed to be activated in extreme crisis, but a lot of us live in crisis all the time. We're in this constant cycle of "I have to get this done or I'll lose my job!" or "I have to get the kids to school, and then I have to clean the house, and why is everything dirty, and I have to cook, and go to the grocery and…" or "I don't have time for this, get the *$%^& out of my way!" (Don't act like you don't know what I'm talking about!)

Adrenal glands compensate for the massive adrenaline onslaught by pumping out a matching amount of cortisol to counterbalance it. This means you get a combination of symptoms of too much adrenaline (high blood pressure, emotional volatility and irritability), and too much cortisol (high blood sugar, tending toward metabolic syndrome and diabetes, weight gain especially in the trunk area, insomnia, and recurrent infections—since your immune system is suppressed). Too much cortisol also inhibits the conversion of inactive to active thyroid hormone, which can lead to hypothyroidism.

After this process goes on for awhile—and how long depends on the person—your adrenals can't keep up with the demand for either adrenaline or cortisol, at which point you feel apathetic and all you want to do is stare at the wall. People who reach this point tend to keep themselves going by drinking massive amounts of caffeine (which indirectly stimulates release of adrenaline—this is essentially like whipping a wounded horse so he'll work harder.) They feel better at first, due to the release of adrenaline… but without the corresponding cortisol to counterbalance it, they crash afterwards (usually with hypoglycemia and sugar cravings) and need more stimulants to keep going.

Lack of sufficient cortisol (which, remember, is anti-inflammatory) also leaves you much more susceptible to allergies, both food and environmental. And it means you don't have enough energy reserves left over to do things like repair tissues, or help your organs of elimination to do their jobs. This can lead to poor wound healing, and chemical sensitivity, too.

Your adrenals also produce a hormone called aldosterone. Aldosterone causes the kidneys to reabsorb sodium and secrete potassium, and water always follows sodium, which means your blood volume increases, which means your blood pressure increases.

Too much chronic stress leads to overworked adrenals in general, so both the adrenaline and the aldosterone output can lead to hypertension.

In the later stages of adrenal fatigue, it's more common to see low blood pressure with adrenal fatigue. That's because they're not pumping out enough aldosterone either. These people will feel the room go dark when they stand up too quickly, and it'll take a second for their vision to catch up to their heads.

Your adrenals also produce a hormone called DHEA. This is the precursor for both the estrogens (estrone, estradiol, and estriol) and testosterone. It's a secondary source of estrogens for women (at least until menopause) and a primary source of testosterone for women. Likewise, DHEA is a secondary source of testosterone for men and a primary source of estrogen.

This is one reason why women who have been under a lot of stress in their pre-menopausal years have such a hard time in menopause: their adrenals are toast. They can't compensate. Menstruating women with adrenal fatigue will also have a lot of trouble with PMS, because at menses, sex hormones drop (that's what causes the shedding of the uterine lining). If you don't have enough DHEA to compensate for this, you'll probably have a lot of issues with PMS, too.

DHEA also counterbalances cortisol. While cortisol suppresses the immune system, thins the skin, and breaks down bone, DHEA bolsters and builds up all of these, encouraging tissue repair. (Testosterone is considered "anti-aging" for a reason.) While cortisol suppresses the thyroid, DHEA also revs up metabolism. So hypothyroidism secondary to adrenal fatigue will improve as cortisol drops and DHEA increases.

If you're not already in adrenal fatigue, you can avoid the whole situation just be learning how to minimize the amount of stress that you cause yourself, and properly dealing with the unavoidable stressors that remain. Even if you are already in adrenal fatigue, learning new strategies to deal with your stress plays an integral part of reversing it. Again, more on adrenal support in Chapter 16.

Reducing Stress Through Time Management

The first thing you can do to reduce the amount of stress in your life is to make a list of your goals.

Separate them into personal and professional areas, and within each category, separate those into long and short term goals. Personal goals might be things like getting in shape, spiritual growth, spending time with family and friends, or learning an instrument. Professional goals might be (for a small business owner like myself) developing a marketing plan, or enforcing one that is already in place. Or it might be studying a new topic that will enhance your career options down the line, or keeping up with professional literature. You know how they say, "If you aim at nothing, you'll hit it every time?" The first step to reaching your goals is always to make them explicit.

Make a list of priorities for each day, and keep it short. If everything is a priority, then nothing is. A list, even one you have created yourself, keeps you from the moment-by-moment crisis of wondering which task to attend to first. If the priorities aren't immediately apparent to you, just pick something. Write it down, and stick to it. Cross off the tasks as you complete them, so that you can see that you're making progress.

Once you know what your priorities are, structure your time to attend to them. Time that isn't structured often ends up being wasted. Stick to one task at a time and complete it in bite-sized intervals. While attending to a task, though, it's important to do your best to prevent distractions. Close Facebook. Close GoogleChat. Close your email. If it's an option, turn off your phone. Structure time at regular intervals to check email and voicemail, and only do it during those allotted times.

Tools like this keep me focused so that I don't waste time, and they also force me to incorporate my personal goals into my routine. Otherwise I'd always find myself doing whatever seemed to be most important in the moment, and before I knew it, all my personal goals would fly right out the window.

At the same time, it's possible to be too structured. I make a point to not create a to-do list one day a week (usually Saturdays), and not on vacation.

Another tip that I find really helpful: get up early. There are a lot fewer distractions in the morning than there are later in the day. Usually nobody expects you to be anywhere or to do anything early in the morning, which makes possible many of your personal goals which might otherwise never happen. I get up at least two hours before I have to leave for the day (before I have to *leave*, not before I have to *arrive*). That way I can wake up, work out, shower, make a healthy breakfast and lunch, spend time in prayer and reading my Bible, and (depending on the day) sometimes work towards a few other goals, like reading professional literature, writing fiction, or responding to personal emails.

It can be difficult to consistently accomplish all that you set out to do in a day, so it is best to create a margin. I've learned this the hard way—if you have literally every moment scheduled with no buffer in between, that's a perfect recipe for stress, because in the real world, nothing ever goes quite the way we planned. Leave room for the accident on the freeway that slows traffic down. For the unanticipated phone call. For a friend to ask you for a favor. The proper ratio is about 80/20—schedule only 80% of your time with either personal, family, or professional goals, and leave 20% available for "life" to happen. If you start to notice that 80% creeping up to 90% or 95%, it might be time to reevaluate whether some of your current goals really need to happen now, or whether they might be better saved for a different season in your life.

Don't forget to schedule time for yourself every day, and guard it. Treat this time like an appointment. It's not negotiable. Try not to set too many expectations for this time, either, or it may become just another "task"—if you spend half an hour just staring at the wall at first, that's fine! The point is just to slow down. Eventually, you will fill the time with activities that you look forward to every day. Remember, it is your responsibility to take care of yourself—nobody is going to do it for you.

Ultimately you are the steward of your time, and it is never worth it to allow yourself to get out of peace. If that happens, the answer is not anti-anxiety medication so that you can maintain your unhealthy breakneck pace… it's to treat the cause!

Of course, it's not possible to remove all of the stressors in your life through time management. There will always be other issues that we have to deal with. For those other stressors, the best thing that we can do is just learn how to manage our stress by properly caring for ourselves physically, mentally, and spiritually.

Reducing Stress Through Lifestyle

I know this is sounding like a reprise of the first half of the book—but one of the most important aspects of stress management is getting enough sleep. Adequate sleep contributes to overall well being, including but not limited to improved energy and greater emotional stability. Not only does sleep help to improve your memory (due to neuroplasticity, the process by which new information is consolidated in your brain during sleep), it also improves performance at whatever you do. This latter benefit is likely due to the fact that during waking hours, a byproduct of neuronal activity called adenosine builds up, leading to fatigue and exhaustion. (Just as a reminder, caffeine works by blocking the effects of adenosine… but only short term.) Sleep gives your body time to clear out the "debris," as it were, and make way for a new day.

Eating a healthy diet is also helpful. High sugar, high saturated fat, and nutrient deficiencies can all cause inflammation and physiologic stress response in your body. Certain nutrients, especially B vitamins, are necessary for the production of neurotransmitters. However, B vitamins are found in dark leafy greens (not exactly a staple of the Standard American Diet) and whole grains (but not white flour, which has been stripped of nutrients). Not only does white flour lack B vitamins of its own, it actually depletes them during the process of digestion. On top of that, white flour and sugar both lead to a glucose spike and subsequent crash, which also sets you up for fatigue and irritability. So eat your complex carbs: veggies, fruit, and whole grains, along with plenty of protein and healthy fats.

Take a fish oil supplement. Essential Fatty Acids increase transmission of neurotransmitters, inhibit the death of brain cells, improve communication of cell membranes (which are sort of the "brains" of your cells), and decrease inflammation. Everybody needs to be taking fish oil. Just make sure you get a good one—they're not all created equal! Refer back to my recommendations on Essential Fatty Acids in Chapter 2.

Make time to exercise regularly. Once again, exercise elevates your mood by releasing endorphins (the natural "high") and improves your metabolism. Exercise is the most potent natural antidepressant there is! It induces production of neurotransmitters that elevate mood, and increases blood flow to both muscles and the brain. Increased blood flow also increases delivery of nutrients and oxygen to those tissues, and eliminates waste products, faster than would happen at rest. (This is important because toxic accumulation can also cause a physiologic stress response.) If you don't have time to hit the gym for an hour every day, simply incorporate movement into your day at regular intervals.

It is also important to maintain a positive attitude as much as possible. Thoughts easily become habits —negative meditation (or worry) produces a negative attitude, and positive meditation does the opposite. Just like any other habit, it's difficult to break the tendency to think negatively at first, but it becomes easier with practice. Be selective about the ideas that you allow to influence your mind. As far as you are able, surround yourself with positive people and up-lifting media (books, music, movies, podcasts, and the like), and shut off those voices that are negative or harmful. It still won't be easy at first to change habits of negative thinking, but this will certainly help to set you up for success.

Practicing effective communication is another important way of managing stress. Many stressful events in our lives come about as a result of poor communication, leading to tension in relationships. Diffuse these situations at the outset as much as possible by speaking truth, in order to avoid larger problems later on.

Remember that leisure activities are an important part of your health and relaxation, too. Consider joining a social or volunteer group with similar interests to yours. Schedule time to get away for the weekend, go on vacation, or spend time with people you love.

Remember that every human has a need to connect with others. One of the most powerful ways to reassure yourself that there's nothing "wrong with you" is to talk to others in a similar circumstance. That's one of the reasons that support groups work so well. The Bible says that we are designed to carry each other's burdens (although each is supposed to carry his own "load", Galatians 6:2-5), implication being that while a load is small enough that we can handle it ourselves, a burden is too large to shoulder alone. Helping, cooperative workplaces or groups promote positive emotions and interdependence, rather than codependence.

Despite all the work you do to keep yourself from becoming stressed, there will be times that stress creeps up on you. It is important to have a regular practice in place to help you relax.

Relaxation Techniques

My favorite relaxation techniques are effective mostly because they are easy to do and can be incorporated into your routine fairly simply. Notice that all of the techniques I present to you involve a shift in focus—that is the key.

Prayer is definitely #1 for me. The idea that we are in control of our own lives is an illusion anyway. Prayer reminds us to place our focus not on the problem, but on the One who can lead us to the solution. Pray about your concerns, but then *be still and listen*. It's a conversation, not a monologue. You'll notice that the more you deal with your ADT (Attention Deficit Trait) by cutting back and slowing down, the easier it will be for you to hear the Holy Spirit speaking back to you. Also, the more you renew your mind with scripture (Romans 12:2), the easier it will become to tell the difference between Him and your own thoughts.

Along those lines, **meditation** is the art of clearing your mind and focusing intently on a single image, phrase, or idea. Worry involves the constant focus on a negative thought or idea, while meditation is the intentional focus on a positive idea. Meditating on scripture is the most effective way to renew your mind with God's faith-filled words, rather than your worries. More on this in Chapter 9.

Use guided imagery. When you worry, you are using your imagination to envision a negative outcome. Why not use the powerful tool of your mind in order to achieve the opposite effect? There are many terrific guided imagery CDs that can help you with this technique if you are not yet adept at creating powerful images on your own.

Develop a yoga practice. This form of slow, methodical stretching holds each pose long enough to release stored tension in the muscles that are forced to relax. It also emphasizes proper breathing.

Deep breathing is a quick way to bring your body into a parasympathetic (or a "not stressed") state. When muscles are tense, they seize up, inhibiting blood flow and oxygenation. Deep breathing provides more oxygen to your tissues, helping to release that tension. Breathe in and out to a count of five seconds each, expanding your stomach rather than your chest. This drops your diaphragm, fills your lungs to capacity, and slows your heart rate.

If none of the other techniques have completely done the trick, get a massage. Ask your partner or pay for a professional when needed. Massage techniques force blood flow back into tense muscles, which both delivers oxygen and whisks away toxins that have stagnated in the tissues.

Summary:

If you have the ability to make changes to mitigate your stress, by all means, do so! But all of us encounter stressful situations that are not under our control. Cultivate a stress management technique, or several, that work for you in order to spare your body some of the toxic physiologic effects of long-term stress.

CHAPTER 14

Obstacle to Cure #5: Prolonged Poor Treatment —> An Unhealthy Gut

If the microbes that make up our gut flora are out of balance, our health will suffer. This includes things like IBD (Irritable Bowel Disease), but it also affects our energy levels, weight, moods and overall mental health, and our immune and nervous systems. There is a wealth of evidence that shows many autoimmune conditions and degenerative disorders are actually rooted in gut dysfunction.

Like the other things we have discussed, our gut health is something that we have control over. If we care for ourselves properly, we can prevent gut dysbiosis (microbial imbalance). If it is too late for that and you are already suffering, there are steps that can be taken to begin healing your body and restoring your microbiome.

Candidiasis

Candidiasis, or Candida (yeast) overgrowth, happens because your gut has its own microscopic ecosystem that needs to stay in balance. Everyone has a trace amount of candida in their guts, but these little guys are opportunists. That means that they don't play offense, but as soon as the good bacteria get wiped out (by a hefty round of antibiotics, say), they will proliferate and fill in the empty space. Nature abhors a vacuum (so said Aristotle).

Candida is a single-celled fungus, or a yeast, and it eats sugar. I tend to think of this when people tell me they're addicted to sugar, or when a diet diary shows me they're eating either a lot of sugar or white carbs (which are essentially the same thing). Because candida eats sugar, people with candidiasis crave it. In a vicious cycle, they'll eat lots of sugar, triggering the pancreas to release a bolus of insulin. Then sugar rushes out of the bloodstream and into the cells, and blood sugar crashes. This leads to shakes and irritability, a condition called hypoglycemia—and even more sugar cravings.

As a byproduct of its sugar metabolism, candida

produces acetaldehyde, the same toxic byproduct your liver produces when processing alcohol. (Acetaldehyde is actually the chemical responsible for hangovers.) So effectively, candida can make you feel a little bit drunk! People usually describe it as poor memory, fuzzy thinking, or poor word recall. Acetaldehyde can also lead to headaches.

Because candida ferments the sugar you eat, you also tend to end up with gas and bloating. One of the byproducts of fermentation is carbon dioxide which, as you can probably imagine, is great in your lungs, but pretty unpleasant in your gut.

Sometimes, when candida overgrowth gets really out of hand, a patient will have yeast issues on their skin. You may recognize this as jock itch, a yeast infection, athlete's foot, ringworm, intertrigo, or thrush. Often a patient will end up itching at some other body orifice, often the ears or throat.

When candida overgrowth gets out of control, it ends up irritating the gut lining, and over time this can cause inflammation. If the inflammation is severe enough, it can lead to food molecules prematurely coming in contact with the bloodstream, and this can trick your body into thinking the food is a foreign invader. This causes food allergies and sensitivities, and can complicate treatment a bit, but it's not at all uncommon.

* * *

Candida overgrowth is definitely one of the conditions I see most frequently, and it's fun to treat because when there aren't any other complicating factors (such as SIBO, leaky gut, mold exposure, etc) then the results are dramatic after about 6 weeks. I very often hear patients tell me, "I didn't even know it was possible to feel this good!"

Food Allergies

Food allergies are incredibly common these days. This is the first thing I think of when I see recurrent sinusitis or upper respiratory infections, asthma, ear infections, GERD or reflux, eczema, or psoriasis. In addition to those, though, food allergies can also cause chronic gut issues (gas, bloating, IBS), fluid retention, autoimmunity, behavioral changes (lots of ADD/ADHD kids do much better when allergens are removed), and I've even seen cases where food sensitivities are responsible for hypertension and weight gain. Circuitously though, food allergies and sensitivity can also stem from a leaky gut that was caused by microbial dysbiosis of some kind. It can turn into a chicken-or-egg type of situation!

Nobody is really sure why food allergies are so prevalent, but there are a few theories that make sense to me.

Food allergies could stem from a lack of beneficial flora (probiotics) in our diets. As mentioned in Chapter 3, probiotics are important because they feed on the waste left over after we digest our food, and produce lactic acid, which helps protect our guts against pathogens. We used to get plenty of them by eating raw and fermented foods... but these days, our food is so processed and overheated that there are precious few good flora left over. And that sets us up for overgrowth by the bad flora.

Medicines that wipe out gut flora are also suspected of causing allergies. These include antibiotics, certainly, but they also include proton pump inhibitors (such as omeprazole), nSAIDs (like ibuprofen), steroids (like prednisone), birth control, and many others.

It has also been suggested that genetically modified foods, as mentioned in Chapter 10, may cause food allergies. This could be because the toxins produced by these foods kill off our gut flora, or because the novel components themselves are stimulating our immune systems.

Really, though, anything causing inflammation in the gut is capable of causing food allergies. This can be a bout of gastroenteritis, trauma, untreated malabsorption syndromes, environmental toxicity, and even chronic stress. If there's inflammation in the lining of the small intestines for any reason, it sets you up to develop sensitivities to foods you could otherwise consume with no problem.

Most people think of allergy testing as a skin-prick test, but this isn't the test I prefer. This is because skin-prick tests identify IgE antibodies only. IgE antibodies cause immediate hypersensitivity reactions, and while this is very useful to know (it may keep you out of the hospital!), it will miss a good 90% of food sensitivities. This is because most food sensitivities trigger IgG antibodies, which have a 72 hour window in the body. This means you can eat something to which you are sensitive, and not react to it for a few days!

IgG testing is a blood test, and it's never covered by insurance, unfortunately. But for patients who aren't able or willing to do the elimination diet (which is as cheap as your grocery bill, but it's a pain), the blood test is definitely worth it. The serum test I use also checks for IgE antibodies to foods at the same time. Every so often I will also do IgA testing, the immunoglobulin specific to the gut itself, or MRT testing, which tests for the release of inflammatory cytokines in response to exposure to a particular food, though it does not necessarily produce immunoglobulins against the food.

Six year old Eliot came to me with chronic skin hives that left pigmented spots all over his body, as well as asthma when he was exposed to the cold. As is the case with almost any chronic skin condition, as well as chronic asthma, I immediately thought food allergies, and we did a finger prick food allergy test. When the results came back, we removed the food allergies that came up, and also gave Eliot glutamine to heal up his gut lining, and probiotics to help restore the integrity of the immune system in his gut. Six weeks later, his skin had mostly cleared up and continued to improve, and his asthma was gone.

Small Intestine Bacterial Overgrowth

Small Intestine Bacterial Overgrowth (called SIBO) occurs when there is a change in the numbers and types of bacteria in the bowel. These changes occur from genetic bowel disorders, antibiotics (killing off the good bacteria and leaving behind the pathogens), dysfunctional organs, and as a complication of diabetes. There's a huge correlation between IBS (Irritable Bowel Syndrome) and imbalanced gut flora. In fact, the two almost always go together.

Imagine you step on a thorn: your foot will get pretty irritated, and then the irritation will draw white blood cells to the area to fight the foreign invader. That, by definition, is inflammation.

In the same way, if your gut is irritated, it's also inflamed. There may be some question as to how the inflammation started in the first place, but eventually it becomes a vicious cycle. In a nutshell, the cycle looks like this: inflammation (from autoimmunity, food allergies, pharmaceuticals that wipe out good gut flora, etc) —> mucus —> inability to break down complex carbs —> gas and acid —> more inflammation —> more mucus... and round and round we go. This can also set you up for leaky gut syndrome (more on this in a bit).

Dysbiosis is almost always a side effect of this process. The only real difference between dysbiosis and SIBO is that SIBO means flora that is supposed to stay in the colon has crawled back into the small intestine, while dysbiosis just means imbalance of gut flora (a more general term).

SIBO has the same signs and symptoms as IBS: gas, bloating, abdominal pain and cramps, both constipation and diarrhea (sometimes in the same patient!), and stools ribboned with mucus. But, in addition to the previous symptoms, SIBO can also cause excessive belching, problems digesting fats (because it interferes with bile), low iron levels (the bacteria themselves can consume some of the iron, accounting for this), and acid reflux (because stomach acid serves as an antibiotic in the stomach. And if it is low, as it often is in acid reflux, this can be one of the causes of SIBO. For this reason, prolonged antacid use can set you up for this too). A real telltale sign of small bacterial overgrowth is if probiotics containing inulin or FOS make you gassy, or fiber actually makes your constipation worse.

There are two ways to test for SIBO: endoscopies and breath tests. The small intestine is really hard to reach, though; endoscopies only reach the upper portion of the SI and colonoscopies only reach the bottom portion, leaving a good 17 feet of the small intestine that we can't see without surgery. For that reason, the best way to go is a breath test.

To perform the breath test, you ingest a form of sugar (lactulose or glucose), and a few hours later your breath will reflect a certain amount of hydrogen and/or methane, both byproducts of small bowel overgrowth. The higher these levels, the more overgrowth you have.

I will say that SIBO is one of the trickiest functional GI problems to treat, largely because the treatment (usually the antibiotic Rifaximin and occasionally Neomycin as well, or a high potency garlic extract) tends to lead to improvement but not total remission. Most cases of SIBO require multiple rounds of treatment.

I believe Lydia was the fastest case of SIBO that I've ever seen resolved, and it required two rounds of antibiotics: one with Rifaximin only, and the second breath test showed higher methane producing bacteria than were present the first time, so the second round included both Rifaximin and Neomycin. After that we successfully transitioned her to a full spectrum probiotic to protect against relapse, and she remained on a modified Specific Carbohydrate Diet with good success.

Irritable Bowel Disease

Irritable Bowel Disease is a special case, and needs to be treated as such. IBD includes autoimmune conditions Crohn's and Ulcerative Colitis (UC), both characterized by GI inflammation, and blood and/or mucus in the stool.

The causes of Crohn's and UC are not completely understood (which is essentially the case with all autoimmune conditions). But once the process starts, according to Elaine Gottschall, author of *Breaking the Vicious Cycle,*[1] the cycle goes something like this:

Think of carbs as sugar (which essentially they are—your body converts them into sugar). Your body can absorb simple (single) sugars directly, but complex sugars have to be broken into simple sugars by enzymes, which are found on your intestinal lining, before absorption becomes possible. Then the newly-minted simple sugars can be absorbed.

If complex carbs don't get broken down (for

whatever reason), then they don't get absorbed, and they travel on down through your intestines. Then they come in contact with the bacteria in your gut. These bacteria break down the carbs for you, but they produce two major byproducts: gas (so you feel distended) and acid (which causes inflammation in your intestines). Your body responds to the inflammation by producing mucus to protect itself.

The problem is, the mucus blocks the enzymes in your intestines from coming in contact with other complex carbs you eat. So more complex carbs get turned into gas and acid, producing even more mucus.

Gottschall's answer to breaking the cycle (and my clinical experience) is this: you have to interfere with the cycle at the only place where you have some control. And the only part you are directly in control of is what you eat.

So if you stop eating carbs that require enzymes to break them down (specifically disaccharides: two sugars hooked up to each other, meaning mostly grains and processed or canned carbs), the nasty bacteria in your gut have nothing to eat. So instead of producing gas and acid, they starve and die. Gas and intestinal inflammation decrease; therefore mucus production decreases.

The rest of the gut-healing protocol is very similar to the approach for food allergies. There are almost always a bunch of food allergies secondary to IBD-associated inflammation, and these will also need to be addressed. Eventually you should be able to add disaccharides back into your diet, as long as you don't overdo it and continue to avoid foods you're allergic to (which may exacerbate or perpetuate the inflammation as well).

As a side note, some (not all) of these patients also tend towards depression or anxiety. My theory is that, because some 80% of the serotonin in the body is produced in the gut, inflammatory gut conditions can sometimes trigger mental/emotional imbalances. If this is the sole or primary source of the problem, your mood may also improve as the gut heals.

Patients who come to me with IBD tend to be heavily medicated, exhausted, and discouraged already, so it can be hard to isolate how much is circumstantial and how much is a true neurotransmitter imbalance. This is especially true because I often treat more than one symptom at a time. Janet came to me with Crohn's Disease just after she'd gotten out of the hospital, with terrible joint pain and such severe fatigue that she spent most of her time in bed. We tested her for food allergies, and put her on a modified Specific Carbohydrate Diet (eliminating the foods to which she was sensitive), gave her the nutrients to heal up her gut lining, and also supported her adrenals —after a long bout of chronic illness, the adrenals are almost always toast, which leads to poor stress resiliency at best and hopelessness at worst. Six weeks later, she was like a new person—her bowel movements were normal, no gas and bloating, joint pain resolved, energy dramatically improved, and of course her mood was much better too. Was it circumstances or gut inflammation that had caused the depression in the first place? No idea, but my guess is a little of both.

As you reintroduce foods back into your diet, you many notice that you have sensitivity reactions to certain foods. By far, the two most common culprits are gluten and dairy.

Dairy Sensitivity

Our ancestors have been drinking dairy for generations with no problems—but now, all of a sudden, dairy sensitivity is second only to gluten sensitivity. What happened?

For those with an already sensitive gut, dairy is a very common culprit. There are a few possible reasons why.

Dairy is often full of antibiotics and added hormones. rBGH and rBST are growth hormones given to about one in six dairy cows in the U.S. to increase milk production. These hormones cause inflammation in the cows' breast tissue, augmenting the need for antibiotics. Dairy cows consume about 70% of this nation's antibiotics both for this reason, as well as to offset the unhealthy conditions in which they are maintained.

The reason this is bad news: bacteria are smart. Antibiotics may kill off most of a given strain, but the ones that survive are the ones that are resistant, and then they reproduce… which is the reason why we're having more and more trouble with antibiotic-resistant bacteria these days. Additionally, as you have already learned in Chapter 10, the milk produced by cows treated with these hormones has a higher concentration of insulin-like growth factor 1 (IGF-1), linked to various kinds of hormonal cancers.

Dairy products often have a number of additives. Reduced fat or fat free milk has been processed to strip away the cream, which also removes the fat-soluble vitamins A and D. These vitamins must then be added back (which, again, is why you should be leery of any product that says it is "enriched". This term means that vitamins and minerals that were lost during processing were added back. But if a food needs to be enriched in the first place, it's been processed. Beware!) Some brands of milk also contain gums like carrageenan, which may cause gut irritation. In general, any product that has been chemically processed is more likely to trigger allergic responses than the original, untampered product.

The two allergens in milk likely to provoke a reaction are the sugar (lactose) and the protein (usually casein, but more rarely, whey). Lactose and whey are found primarily in softer milk products, such as milk and ice cream, while casein is found primarily in harder milk products, such as hard cheeses, yogurt, and kefir.

If you suspect you are sensitive to either lactose or casein (or whey), eliminate it for 2 weeks, and then eat a lot of it for three days. If you're sensitive to it, you'll know right away. However, this will only work if dairy is your only sensitivity. If there are more, the picture will be muddier, at which point you would have to do either a full elimination diet, or a blood test.

Gluten Sensitivity

The only thing more prevalent than a sensitivity to dairy is a gluten sensitivity. It's a little weird, right? People have been eating wheat since the agricultural age began, some 10,000 years ago. So why the sudden explosion in Celiac Disease and gluten sensitivity?

Celiac Disease is an autoimmune condition: it means that in response to the presence of gluten, the body produces antibodies that attack the lining of the small intestine, blunting the villi and preventing absorption of nutrients. An autoimmune condition is when your body attacks itself.

If you have Celiac disease, then you'll have to avoid gluten very strictly, and forever.

Gluten sensitivity, on the other hand, is an allergy —it just means the body produces antibodies (IgG or IgE) against the gluten protein, causing inflammation and poor digestion in the gut. An allergy is when your body attacks something that is ordinarily harmless. In this case, the harmless substance is gluten protein which is the glue, or the core binding element, of certain grains (including wheat of course, plus barley, bulgar, couscous, durum, rye, semolina, spelt, and triticale—to name a few).

Nobody really had any issues digesting gluten until around fifty years ago, around the end of World War II. Since then, the rate of Celiac Disease has risen over 400%—and that's to say nothing of the many others who are merely gluten sensitive. There seem to be two possible explanations for this: how we grow and process wheat changed around 1960, and how we get the dough to rise (ferment) changed most significantly during the aforementioned war.

Bread rises due to fermentation. Organisms produce energy from sugar either aerobically (in the presence of oxygen) or anaerobically (oxygen not necessary). Fermentation is an anaerobic process, converting sugar into (in this case) lactic acid and carbon dioxide. The latter is a gas, and that's what makes bread rise.

Up until about a hundred years ago, sourdough was the only kind of bread available, and it is produced in the following manner: flour + water + a sealed container + time –> sourdough starter (consisting of a whole bunch of different strains of bacteria + CO_2 + lactic acid). While the CO_2 makes the bread rise, the lactic acid gives it its characteristic sour flavor. But lactic acid also has three other very important functions: it serves as a natural preservative; it helps to break down certain naturally occurring chemicals (called phytobiotics) that prevent the body from absorbing the nutrients found in the grain; and, most relevant to the topic at hand, lactic acid helps to break down the gluten protein. (Remember, gluten is sticky like glue, and therefore harder to digest on its own, without this assistance.)

Around 1879, however, mass-produced commercial yeast was invented, consisting only of a single strain of yeast (saccharomyces cerevisiae), compared to the veritable zoo of microflora found in sourdough starters. This single yeast ferments the bread much quicker than in sourdough, minimizing or eliminating the benefits of lactic acid. During WWII, this yeast was further refined into granulated active dry yeast, and it was refined further still into instant yeast in the 1970s. (See a correlation in these timelines?)

In 1961, wheat crops also began to be mass-produced. Mass production meant the grain had to be able to withstand fertilizers, pesticides, heavy machinery, and transcontinental shipping... and in order to achieve such hearty grain, the wheat was bred to contain more gluten than ever before. (Remember, gluten is glue—more gluten means it can take more of a beating.) In order to accommodate the extra gluten in the same amount of "space", though, the trace mineral content in wheat correspondingly declined (and that's before commercial processing strips out the rest of it).

If you *are* gluten sensitive (but do not have Celiac) you are left with avoiding all gluten-containing food types or replacing your usual carbohydrate products with gluten-free products. But there is a problem. It is sad, but true... most pre-packaged products marketed as "gluten-free" are still highly processed white carbohydrates, which means the carbs turn into sugar as soon as they hit your saliva (which is a problem for a variety of reasons). You might not have an allergic response to it, but that doesn't make it nutritious.

The good news, though, is that by following traditional grain preparation methods, gluten-containing grains may be tolerable!

In 2007, Applied and Environmental Microbiology performed a study demonstrating that while ordinary wheat bread contains gluten levels of 75,000 parts per million, its fermented (sourdough) counterpart instead contained only 12 parts per million—rendering it effectively gluten-free.

Sprouting your grains is another way to achieve essentially the same effect. Raw food naturally contains probiotics and enzymes—enzymes which do essentially the same thing that lactic acid does in terms of breaking down the gluten protein for you. Ezekiel is my favorite brand of sprouted grain products, although you can certainly sprout your own, if you have the time and inclination.

If you have Celiac Disease, you still need to avoid even sourdough or sprouted grains. But even some of my most gluten-sensitive patients can tolerate sourdough and sprouted grains with no problems.

As a medical student, I got food allergy tested and found out I was allergic to almost everything! Gluten was on the list, and as I paid more attention, I noticed that I developed eczema, bloating, and itching a few days after I consumed it. Now that I've healed up my gut lining, I still employ a rotation diet, such that I only consume gluten-containing grains in large quantities at most every three days; but I can have 100% sourdough or Ezekiel bread daily and suffer no ill effects from it.

Healing Your Gut

The bottom line with microbial overgrowths and food allergies is that you have to heal your gut.

If you suffer from Candidiasis, you need to cut out the sugar. Also cut out the white carbs (which are the same thing), as well as any other yeasts, fungi, or fermented foods (like vinegar and alcohol). You can add back the latter eventually, but it's a good idea to always keep sugar and white carbs to a minimum!

You should also take steps to actually kill the candida that is present. There are some excellent over-the-counter antifungal products, but garlic is one of the most potent of all—and you can cook with it!

Finally, you need to repopulate your gut with health-promoting microbes. Find a probiotic with a 50/50 ratio of bifidobacillus to lactobacillus, and at least 20 billion organisms per day.

This process is straightforward, but it's not easy, especially if you're addicted to sugar. Give it six weeks, though, and you'll be amazed at how much better you feel.

But for most patients who show up with IgG food sensitivities secondary to gut inflammation, stress, or low beneficial gut flora, it only takes about six weeks to heal up the gut lining. During that time you'll need to avoid the foods you're sensitive to while we heal up your gut, but after that you can begin adding back most of the foods to which you were reactive—in moderate amounts. However, any food that had a very high IgG titer will have to remain an occasional treat only, rather than a regular part of your diet. (After six weeks, most people feel so much better that they have no desire to return to their previous diets anyway!)

CHAPTER 15

Obstacle to Cure #6: Prolonged Poor Treatment
—> A Confused Immune System

Your immune system's job is to keep you healthy, but sometimes it gets a little confused and produces an unbalanced antibody population, or even antibodies that are ultimately harmful. Autoimmune conditions and allergies both result from those mistaken antibodies.

There are two parts to your immune system, called non-specific (this responds right away to toxic exposure, bee stings, trauma, etc) and specific (which takes some time, but is more targeted against specific invaders). Think of non-specific immunity like a sledge hammer, while specific immunity is more like a scalpel. The sledge hammer is quick and dirty, and (as you might imagine) will cause a lot of inflammation even in surrounding healthy tissues. The scalpel, on the other hand, won't cause as much collateral damage, but it will have to be very carefully directed in order to do any good.

Because your **specific immune system** (the scalpel) needs careful direction, two kinds of cells are necessary: the T and B cells.

If I can mix my metaphors, think of the T cells as the managers and the B cells as the worker bees (no pun intended)—that is, the B cells actually produce antibodies against specific invaders, while the T cells tell the B cells what to do.

Now there are three types of substances (called antigens) that have the potential to provoke your *specific immune system* to make antibodies against them. There are soluble antigens (these come from your diet and your environment), insoluble antigens (these come from microbes and pathogens), and self antigens (these come from your own cells).

Reactions against soluble antigens are called allergies.

Reactions against self antigens are called autoimmune diseases.

Reactions against insoluble antigens is normal immune function.

Those T and B cells that produce the wrong kinds

of antibodies are supposed to be destroyed before they ever enter the bloodstream, but since some get out anyway, there's a built in checks-and-balances system: the Regulatory T cells.

Fortunately, Regulatory T cells are produced in proportion to the number of rogue immune cells (mixing metaphors one more time: if you have more criminals, you need more cops). But your gut can also produce Regulatory T cells under the right set of conditions. In fact, 80% of your immune system is in your gut. This makes sense, doesn't it? After all, your gut is your body's first line of defense, since that's where your organs first come in contact with the outside world.

So, with both allergic and autoimmune patients of almost any diagnosis, I usually start with the gut (and if I don't start with it, I always address it at some point). The goal is to a) produce more Regulatory T cells (more cops) to stop the antibodies against self or soluble antigens (criminals), and b) to increase the production of antibodies against insoluble antigens—the true foreign invaders.

Elaine, a 55 year old artist, came to me in my first year of practice with a diagnosis of Rheumatoid Arthritis. The joint pain was a big problem for her especially, because her job required her to use her hands. She had quite a few food allergies and environmental allergies as well. After "retraining" her immune system with the sublingual al-

lergy spray for the environmental sensitivities, elimination of food allergies, and healing her gut lining, today she comes to see me just for the occasional cold of bout of fatigue. No joint pain!

Back to the sledgehammer (non-specific immunity): in the case of both autoimmune and allergic patients, although it's the specific immunity that's gone awry (the scalpel is targeting the wrong things), the sledgehammer tries to pick up the slack. As a result, there's always a lot of inflammation going on in these patients too. My first approach is to identify and remove sources of inflammation, ensuring a good diet that's chock-full of anti-inflammatory oils and antioxidants. It's of course very helpful to also reduce exposure (in the case of allergies) to decrease this inflammatory response when possible. When exposure is unavoidable, we may try to build an immune tolerance instead, using very small but increasing exposure to the antigen (with a sublingual allergy spray—like shots, but without the needle).

Allergies

Your immune system is designed to protect your body against harmful substances, such as bacteria, viruses, and foreign substances (allergens). In that sense, allergic responses are not inherently bad. But in a person with allergies, the immune response is exaggerated, and you react to substances that are not generally harmful.

The word "allergies" is kind of a catch-all term, since it can refer to allergic conjunctivitis, atopic dermatitis (eczema), contact dermatitis, hay fever (seasonal allergies), or food or drug allergies, which tend to manifest symptoms all over the body. As mentioned in Chapter 14, allergies pretty much always go back to the gut.

Common allergens include drugs, dust, food (these can be to the protein, starch, additive, or pesticide on the food), insect bites, mold, pet dander, pollen, hot or cold temperatures, sunlight, or other environmental triggers. Sometimes even friction can cause symptoms in highly reactive individuals.

There are actually five kinds of antibodies in your body, but for the purposes of allergy testing, we only care about three: IgE, IgA, and IgG. IgE are considered "immediate sensitivity" antibodies, which means your body mounts an immune response to that substance immediately. IgG are "delayed sensitivity" antibodies, which means it may take your body up to 72 hours to mount an immune response. IgA are the antibodies that are specific to your gut lining.

Skin prick tests are the most common method of allergy testing, and the one conducted in most allergists' offices. This measures IgE ("immediate sensitivity" antibodies). Blood tests can measure either IgE, or IgG. Food allergies are best measured with IgG antibody blood tests, because 80-95% food reactions are of the IgG variety. Blood tests for IgE antibodies are more valuable for environmental allergens such as molds, pet dander, pollens, grasses, dust and the like. (These usually are covered by most insurance policies, but sometimes you have to fight for it.)

The traditional approach to treating allergies is with suppressive medication. Most medications for allergies focus on symptom relief, including antihistamines, steroids, decongestants, and a few other medicines that work by different mechanisms (such as Singulair). Although these medicines can be effective for many patients, they do not address the root cause of immune system hypersensitivity, and side effects can be prohibitive.

For severe allergies or allergens that cannot be avoided, shots are often recommended. These work much like vaccines, exposing your body to a small amount of each allergen at a time so that it "gets used to" it. They work well for some patients, but they require frequent (usually weekly) trips to the doctor.

The primary approach in traditional medicine is the same as in naturopathic medicine (at least initially), and that is the avoidance of triggers. This is important while we figure out what else is causing the hypersensitivity reactions and address the root cause.

After that, it's always important to start by cleaning up your diet. You need adequate nutritional support in order to heal, or at least to avoid undue stress on your system that will impede healing.

Allergies of any kind almost always involve the gut. This, again, is because 80% of your immune system is in your gut—it produces another antibody, called IgA. Ideally, your gut should produce a lot of IgA, because it's your first line of defense against any foreign substance. (A lot, but not too much.) The flora and the lining of your gut need to be healthy in order to produce adequate IgA so that the rest of your body never has to deal with those substances. My most common go-to is glutamine, the food for the lining of your small intestine. I recommend 4-5 grams daily for at least the 6 weeks of initial avoidance, along with some heavy duty probiotics.

Next, it's important to assess whether your adrenals are acting properly. High stress or inflammation leads to a high demand for a hormone called cortisol, and this can also decrease production of IgA. More on this in Chapter 16.

Next, you must assess your liver. People with allergies often have a high toxic body burden. Toxins are foreign substances which really are harmful to your body (unlike allergens which are not—see Chapter 11), and they need to be altered in some way so that your body can eliminate them. This alteration usually happens in the liver. When there are too many toxins and your liver can't keep up, these toxic substances build up in the system. This may increase reactivity to substances that would ordinarily be considered harmless.

Angela was a 21 year old college student who came to me with severe joint and abdominal pain, chronic weight loss, diarrhea, multiple chemical sensitivities, and insomnia. All of her symptoms began both when she moved into a moldy house, and when she went to a third world country around the same time—so it was unclear to us which was the trigger. At the first visit, we put her on cholestyramine for the mold, performed a stool culture to assess for parasites, and did food allergy testing. We also started adrenal support for irritability and fatigue.

It turned out that Angela did not have parasites, but she did have yeast overgrowth, hemolytic E coli overgrowth, and elevated secretory IgA suggestive of inflammation. Food allergies also showed sensitivity to dairy, gluten, buckwheat, eggs, mushrooms, sugar, and yeast. My suspicion is that her trip to Mexico led to the E coli overgrowth, which caused inflammation and leaky gut, and that yeast overgrew subsequently.

After a 6 week combined allergy elimination and yeast elimination protocol, and a potent garlic extract to kill of the E. coli, Angela returned with all of her symptoms resolved. I believe it was necessary to treat not only her allergies, but the other complicating factors all at once to restore balance.

The Effects of Stress on the Immune System

Allergies and autoimmune diseases get worse when you're stressed, due to low amounts of cortisol. Most allergens stimulate the release of inflammatory substances like histamine. Lack of sufficient cortisol (which, remember, is anti-inflammatory) means you can't naturally suppress these reactions. So while you may always have had a sensitivity to a particular substance (food or environmental), it's not until your body loses its ability to manufacture enough of the naturally anti-inflammatory cortisol that you start to notice them.

If you're super stressed, you're likely to also have more allergies and/or autoimmune activity than you used to. But it's a catch-22: if you have allergies and autoantibodies, you've got inflammation. Inflammation stresses your adrenals, forcing them to produce more cortisol to counterbalance it. So even if you don't have adrenal fatigue to begin with, the longer you struggle with allergies and/or autoimmune disease, the more likely you are to develop adrenal fatigue as a result.

Chronic Viral Infections

Lauren Deville

Chronic viral infections also deplete our immune systems and lead to problems with allergies and autoimmune antibodies.

Your immune system can fight off and eradicate most viral infections, but certain viruses never completely disappear. This is because they hide out in your cells, dormant, waiting to be reactivated.

Viruses work by using your own cellular machinery against you. They latch on to the cell membrane, insert their DNA (or RNA) into the cell, and hijack the cell to manufacture its proteins for it. Even worse, your immune system won't know to attack because from the outside, nothing abnormal is going on. Viruses in the Herpes family (Epstein Barr Virus, Human Herpes Virus 6, Herpes Simplex 1 and 2, and Cytomegalovirus) fall under this category.

In most cases, infection with these viruses is not a big deal, because they are not particularly virulent—for instance, by around age 40, 95% of the population has been infected with Epstein Barr (EBV), but most of them never know it. A robust immune system can keep the virus in check.

Certain triggers, however, can cause sleeping viruses to wake up again. Reactivation triggers include superinfection with another virus (for instance, HHV-6 can trigger reactivation of EBV); trauma to the nerve where the virus resides; stress or physical trauma; and immune system suppression (from chronic illness, autoimmunity, toxic burdens, lack of sleep, poor diet, etc).

When you first get infected with a virus, your body makes an immunoglobulin called IgM specific to that virus to fight it off. These stay elevated only for the first 6-12 weeks; so if you suspect the infection is that new, this would be the one to look for.

After that period of time, the IgM numbers (think of these as your first line of defense) will die down to zero, and instead you'll have elevated IgG (think of these as the reserves). These can tell you that you either have an active chronic infection, or that you had a past infection and the reserves are sticking around to make sure nobody gets out of hand again.

There isn't really a definitive way to tell whether the elevated IgG numbers are due to an active or a past infection, unfortunately. Typically I look for titer numbers to determine this: very high antibody counts suggest that active recruitment is still happening, because the invaders aren't gone. You can also check for the DNA of the invader: high DNA material indicates that the virus is replicating.

No matter what the cause of your immune problems, it is important to support your immune system with nourishing foods. Diet either reduces or creates inflammation; there really isn't a middle ground. The food you eat makes a difference in your ability to fight off infections or normalize antibodies!

Ed is a 70 year old exceptionally pleasant man—he's always polite and cheerful, even when describing his health ailments. About 15 years ago, he got sick with a low grade fever and just never recovered, managing the achiness and malaise with high and continuous narcotics. Even then he usually felt under the weather. He brought me a stack of chart notes and labs that dated through the years, with nearly every type of specialist, but he'd still defied diagnosis.

Initially I suspected that Ed had a chronic viral infection. Sure enough, his lab work came back with high HHV-6 titers. Because of the length of the infection, we also tested cortisol levels (the stress hormone, which also suppresses the immune system). This too was elevated.

After a few months of treatment for both of these along with some diet modifications, Ed managed to wean off of narcotics. The challenge now is maintaining his immune function and sticking with a healthier diet!

Foods that Support the Immune System

Did you know that a little bit of excess sugar in your bloodstream can shut down your immune function for up to 4 hours at a time? If you have problems with your immune system, it is vital to include foods

335

from some key nutrient categories to make sure you're functioning at optimal level.

You should aim to eat protein at every meal and with every snack. Proteins, remember, are made of amino acids, and amino acids are the building blocks for just about every part of your body, including antibodies. (If you lack the bricks, you're not gonna have much of a building!) Whole food protein sources include grass-fed meat, soy (non-GMO of course), dairy, quinoa, beans, eggs, fish, nuts, and nut butters.

Adequate intake of all vitamins and minerals is also critical. Your immune system is complex, so all of the vitamins (both fat and water soluble) are necessary. It's best to get these from food sources, rather than from supplements, because that will ensure the proper balance between them. Multivitamins usually also contain the proper ratios, and I suggest that you take them just to fill in any gaps.

The vitamin everyone thinks of for immune support is **Vitamin C,** and it is very beneficial as an antioxidant, and also helps to generate certain immune cells. Your body burns through more of it than usual in times of stress, illness or otherwise, so it's good to get in more. Great sources include citrus fruits, as well as peppers, broccoli, and other greens. Be careful of the proverbial orange juice, though—while it's high in Vitamin C, juices are also high in sugar.

All of the **B vitamins** are also in higher demand during times of stress, physical or otherwise, and are likewise necessary for generation of immune cells. Dark leafy greens are my favorite food source of B vitamins, but whole grains and cruciferous vegetables such as cauliflower, broccoli, brussels sprouts and cabbage are also good sources of several of them. B12 exists in quantity only in animal products —meat, organ meat, fish, and eggs.

My secret weapon for acute illness is **Vitamin A**. The World Health Organization has used high doses for short periods of time (a few days to a week) for acute illness for some time. I recommend using it in high doses only under the supervision of a licensed physician, however, as it is possible to overdose (generally producing a nasty headache), and it is contraindicated in pregnancy at high doses. Food sources of Vitamin A are the same as those for B12 (meat, organ meat, fish, and eggs), but its water-soluble counterpart, carotenoids, can be found in red, orange, and yellow veggies.

In medical school I discovered the power of high dose Vitamin A, around 150,000 IU daily, and wet socks at the slightest sign of an acute illness. Those two would pretty much knock out anything before it got started!

For wet socks, take two pairs of socks, one thick and wool and one thin and cotton. Before bed, run the thin ones under water and put them in the freezer. Take them out when they're not quite frozen solid, put them on, and put the warm dry thick socks on on top. It'll be unpleasant for the first five minutes, yes—but the hydrotherapy will spike your immune system's production of white blood cells, and will also help your organs of elimination to filter the blood faster than would happen physiologically. I promise they'll be toasty and bone dry by the time you wake up.

Vitamin D, the darling of the nutritional world at the moment, also supports proper immune function. It has been associated with decreased risk of cancer, immune support as well as autoimmune regulation, mood support, and any number of other conditions. Our bodies form active Vitamin D in response to sunlight, but it can also be found in animal food sources, such as milk, fatty fish, and organ meats, as well as (these days) fortified foods. Again, I recommend using it in high doses only under the supervision of a licensed physician, because it is possible to overdose.

Zinc is a mineral involved in nearly every process in the body, but it's especially vital for your T-cells. Since zinc is so necessary for our bodies, it's also abundant in our food—it can be found in various kinds of meat, seafood (like oysters and crab), mustard greens, a variety of nuts and seeds, beans including soy beans, whole grains, and dairy... so basically, if you eat whole food, you can't really avoid it.

A number of other minerals, such as **copper, manganese,** and **selenium,** are also necessary for immune function. Although I prefer food sources of nutrients in general, since our food isn't as nutrient dense as it used to be, I do suggest that all of my patients take a quality multivitamin daily, and that will act as insurance against deficiency.

The best multivitamins contain antioxidants in addition to vitamins and minerals, but no matter what vitamin product you take, it is always critical to make sure you are consuming foods that provide what you need. Colorful fruits and vegetables are rich sources of antioxidants and will generally speed the healing of injured tissues. Keep yourself healthy by eating nutrient-dense, unprocessed foods!

Fasting

Sometimes, even when you are eating all the right foods, it's necessary to really jumpstart your immune function. The best tool for this is fasting. Short fasts (2-4 days) regenerate your immune system in a couple of ways.[1]

While you are fasting, your immune system scales back its production of immune cells. But it also uses this time to "clean house": when you have less energy coming in, it forces your body to be more efficient, which means cutting waste. This includes dismantling older or diseased immune cells.

Once you start eating again, it stimulates your stem cells (those cells in your body that don't know what kind of cell they want to be when they grow up) to become new, healthy immune cells.

Patients undergoing immunosuppressive therapies such as chemotherapy would do well to consider short-term fasts as a supplementary treatment. It also may be an excellent adjunctive treatment for patients suffering from other forms of immune system dysfunction, including autoimmune conditions or even allergies.

Disclaimer: the research on fasting is based on a *complete* fast (as opposed to a juice fast or a cleanse, or a very simple diet). But there are people who shouldn't do a complete fast. Even if you feel that you are a person who can do a complete fast, there are a few guideline that you should keep in mind.

If you are already malnourished, anemic, pregnant, or growing (i.e. a child), a complete fast isn't for you. If you have a wasting disease like cancer, you are also essentially malnourished already and I'd strongly recommend close supervision from a physician, if you try this at all.

If you're going to fast, it's a good idea to prepare

before you start and transition into it by eating lightly for a few days beforehand. This will help to ease the transition.

You will also need to cut back on your daily activities. The more active we are, the more calories we need. If you are restricting (or especially eliminating) your calories, you need to restrict your daily activities as well (and that includes mental activity, too). Don't try a fast on a normal day when you already feel overtaxed.

Especially while fasting, drink *lots* of water. Staying hydrated is always important, but it's critical while fasting, since your body will be detoxing, and you'll need to flush that stuff out of your system.

When you are done, break the fast *slowly*. If you did an extended fast, add one day of transition for every 3-4 days you went without food, and make sure you are choosing simple, natural, easy-to-digest foods such as an apple, steamed veggies, or broth.

Further Immune Support

Although I believe high-quality food (or the absence of food altogether) is the best treatment for a confused immune system, there are a few other things that you can do to restore balance: deal with your energy drainers, get evaluated for adrenal fatigue (both addressed more fully in the next chapter), and possibly get help for chronic viral infections, if applicable.

The natural treatments I recommend for chronic viral infections include coconut oil (or its powerful antiviral extract, monolaurin) and lysine. Lysine is an amino acid that prevents replication of HSV 1 and 2 by inserting itself in place of an amino acid these viruses do require (arginine). It's not known for certain whether it will do the same for all the other viruses in the Herpes family, but I've used it with good clinical results. The dose I recommend is 1 gram daily for maintenance, and 3-4 grams daily for active infection.

The Take-Home Message:

* If you suffer from autoimmunity, allergies, or really any kind of chronic inflammation, **you need food allergy testing**. I recommend IgG immunoglobulins, with total elimination of the offending foods (or at least the highest titer offending foods) completely for 6 weeks, along with nutrients to heal up your gut lining (see Chapter 14).
* If your immune system is weak, I can almost guarantee your adrenals are weak too, because they're very interconnected. **Get a salivary cortisol**

test (and check out Chapter 16).

- Make sure you're **eating real food** (eat the way I suggest at the end of Chapter 1), and **avoid sugar as much as possible**. Sugar is a big, big enemy of your immune system's ability to function at its best.

CHAPTER 16

Obstacle to Cure #7: Prolonged Poor Treatment —> Exhausted Adrenals

When you're stressed out, you don't recover as fast from any kind of stress, including illnesses, hard workouts, or physical traumas like surgery. Here's a quick recap of the stress response.

When something stressful happens, the core of your adrenals flood your body with adrenaline automatically. This makes your heart race, your bronchioles dilate, and provides your muscles with immediate blood flow (oxygen and glucose for energy) to get away quickly or fight, if it comes to that. But even after the situation has calmed down, your body still remains in a state of stress, or high alert. Due to the rush of adrenaline, you've just consumed massive sugar reserves (so now you're probably shaky and hypoglycemic), your blood pressure and heart rate are really high, and your body has totally neglected normal life maintenance stuff like digesting your food and repairing your tissues.

To compensate for these effects of adrenaline, your body releases a hormone called cortisol, which is produced by the outside of your adrenal glands. Cortisol helps to correct the carnage of the adrenaline surge and encourages the breakdown of glycogen (stored glucose) and gluconeogenesis (production of new glucose from fat in the liver). It redirects blood flow to digest food. It's the natural steroid of your body, so it's an anti-inflammatory as well... and also an immune suppressant.

In healthy people, both adrenaline and cortisol will go back to normal levels following an acutely stressful situation. Your body must always have a certain amount of cortisol all the time, and it should start off highest when you wake in the morning, declining throughout the day. A too-high cortisol baseline (due to chronic adrenaline overload) puts you in the Early Stage Adrenal Fatigue category. A too-low cortisol baseline puts you in the Late Stage Adrenal Fatigue category. Both are problematic for immune function and healing.

* * *

Acute (Early Stage) Adrenal Fatigue

The long-term effect of an acutely stressful situation (one that's only started in the last few weeks to few months) is going to be high circulating cortisol, which will suppress your immune function. As anyone who has used topical corticosteroids like hydrocortisone knows, cortisol also thins the skin—and it weakens tissues in general. (This is why cortisone injections may help inflammatory pain in the short-term, but over time will weaken fascia and exacerbate the original problem.)

What this means: if you're in a stressful period in your life, you'll have more anti-inflammatory cortisol circulating to begin with, which increases the chances of getting sick. Then if you do get sick, that's another stressor, requiring initially more adrenaline and then more cortisol to deal with it. Given the amount of your baseline cortisol, you'll have a harder time bouncing back.

Or if you're in that same stressful period and then you have a hard workout, this too will initially spike more adrenaline and then more cortisol... but the higher cortisol "set point" from before the workout will hinder your body's ability to recruit the necessary cytokines to heal the muscle microtears that result from your intense workout.

The very same rules apply to surgery: in itself surgery is a major stressor, and it requires sufficient cortisol to counteract the adrenaline spike. But if you had too much cortisol going into surgery, this will hinder your body's healing process afterwards.

Jennifer is a beautiful 28 year old gym rat; she even competed in bodybuilding competitions. She speaks quickly and with high intensity. She came to me because even at her age, she wasn't making the gains in her workouts that she once did. She felt, given her strict paleo diet and her several-hours-per-day workout routine, she should look more toned than she did, and she should feel more energetic than she did. She also told me that her post-workout recovery time was getting longer, and she'd "hit the wall" much sooner than she ever had before.

What Jennifer described was classic for early stage adrenal fatigue. We did salivary cortisol testing, and found that sure enough, her levels were higher than they should have been thought the day. I put her on a protocol involving not only adaptogenic herbs to support her adrenal function and phosphatidylserine, a lipid derived from sunflowers that helps to blunt excess cortisol, but also sustained release vitamins C and B. These were necessary so that her adrenals could receive a steady dose throughout the day of the nutrients they required for repair. I also gave her a stern talking-to that when she suddenly felt more energy, she should not use that as an excuse to push herself even harder! The fatigue was her body telling her that it needs time to rest and recover, and the only way to prevent a more severe relapse later on would be to listen to it and give it some R&R occasionally. (That's usually the danger with very driven individuals: adrenal fatigue can be your body's signal that you need to "slow down!", while adrenal support can actually be detrimental if you do not heed its warning.)

Late Stage Adrenal Fatigue

Later stages of adrenal stress occur when the adrenals are no longer able to produce enough cortisol to compensate for the adrenaline surges. This stage is usually marked by fatigue, hypoglycemia, low blood pressure, increased allergies as well as environmental and chemical sensitivities, estrogen dominance, and (ironically) poor wound healing—because your body doesn't have enough energy (literally, enough glucose) to perform all its functions efficiently.

Late stage adrenal fatigue also affects many other functions that are not apparently obvious: adrenal problems are often the underlying physiological stress behind hormonal problems and hair loss.

Adrenal Fatigue and Estrogen Dominance

Adrenal fatigue sets you up for estrogen dominance (more on this in Chapter 17). This predisposes women to PMS (irritability, weepiness, anxiety, depression, mood swings), breast tenderness, severe

menstrual cramping; heavy, prolonged bleeding
(menorrhagia), spotting between cycles, thick clotting in menstrual blood, acne, hot flashes and night
sweats, water retention, fibrocystic breasts, fibroids,
migraines, and endometriosis. This is because all of
the adrenal hormones have a common ancestor: cholesterol.

Cholesterol is also the precursor of pregnenolone
and 17-OH-pregnenolone. Those hormones are the
precursors of all of the sex hormones in your body.
They are also the precursors of the adrenal hormones.

Progesterone (the main hormone that counteracts
estrogen) is a precursor in the adrenal glands for both
cortisol and another adrenal hormone, aldosterone
(the one responsible for blood pressure changes).
While estrogen encourages tissue proliferation (i.e.
makes more of your endometrial lining, which can
lead to heavy periods), progesterone does the opposite, nourishing the endometrial lining in case you get
pregnant. (You can remember this if you break the
word down into its constituents: *Pro-Gestation*.) It
also counterbalances the estrogen dominance symptoms above, helping to lift the mood, restore libido,
improve memory, assist with sleep, and protect
against endometrial cancer.

Of the adrenal hormones, cortisol is the most important. Too much is a problem, but too little is disas-

ter. If the body has to choose which of the steroid hormones to make, it'll pick cortisol every time. This means in times of high stress, when we need more cortisol to counterbalance adrenaline, our bodies will pass right on through the progesterone stage and make cortisol.

Erin, 24, came to see me after she'd done a lot of self-healing already. She has a diagnosis of Hashimoto's, or antibodies against her thyroid, and already was on a good dose of compounded T4/T3; she'd been tested for and eliminated a number of food allergies, and she had a history of cramping during her periods so severe that she would sometimes have to go to the ER. All of these symptoms arrived during a time of high stress in her life.

After embarking on a protocol of yoga and meditation in addition to balancing her thyroid and avoiding food allergies, Erin was dramatically better—so much so that her only remaining symptoms were the week before and during her period. At that time, she developed immense fatigue, cramping, gas and bloating, depression, acne breakouts, low blood pressure, and heavy cycles.

I explained to Erin that this was likely because her adrenals had never fully recovered to 100%; they produced just enough cortisol to keep her afloat, as long as she had no additional stressors to contend with. But because cortisol is anti-inflammatory, additional inflammation (such as foods to which she is sensitive) would push her over into symptoms. Likewise, around her cycle, the ovaries dramatically reduce their production of the female sex hormones, and the adrenals must take over, with DHEA. Unfortunately, DHEA and cortisol share the common ancestor of cholesterol—and remember, cortisol is more important. When the body has to pick, it'll pick cortisol every time. Likewise, the direct precursor for cortisol is progesterone... but when the body has to pick, it will shunt the progesterone to cortisol also. These both set her up for symptoms of estrogen dominance, and symptoms of adrenal fatigue—which only occur around her cycle.

Hair Loss due to Adrenal Stress

Hair loss is very common among both men and women, but in different patterns.

Male pattern baldness is usually associated with an excess of dihydrotestosterone (DHT), a metabolite of testosterone in the androgen family. This is genetic, and aside from medications and supplements that block the enzyme which converts testosterone to DHT (called 5-alpha reductase), there isn't much to be done about this one.

Female hair loss often results from autoimmunity, hypothyroidism, or deficiency in the storage form of iron, called ferritin. Women may also suffer from androgenic hair loss, often associated with Polycystic Ovarian Syndrome (PCOS). More on this in Chapter 17.

Then there's a diagnosis called *telogen effluvium*. Essentially this diagnosis means hair falls out due to physiologic stress... or emotional stress which leads to physiologic stress.

Physiologic stress includes things like lack of sleep, improper eating habits, weight gain or loss, hormonal changes, or severe or prolonged illness. Emotional stress may lead to these things, though, as stress hormones have a tendency to produce physiologic changes. But it takes awhile for these physiologic changes to produce a cumulative effect leading to hair loss (3-6 months), so it may be difficult to pinpoint the cause of the hair loss.

If you've ruled out all other causes of hair loss, and you've undergone some major physiologic or emotional changes in the last 3-6 months, it's likely that either physical or emotional stress may be your culprit.

Rachel, 31, came to me with a chief concern of hair loss. For a little while we chased the potential cause—her thyroid was slightly suboptimal but not 'off' enough to really account for the problem. Her ferritin was low, but iron supplementation didn't seem to slow down the problem either.

It wasn't until Rachel really opened up to me about what was going on in her life that the real issue became clear. She came from an abusive family, and she was currently in an abusive relationship—but she had no outlet for her emotions, no one to whom she felt safe enough to share her struggles. She felt guilty all the time, and felt responsible for her parents' ongoing struggles. She wanted to protect her mother from her abusive father, but her mother was unwilling to allow her help.

On her own, Rachel began to take steps to set bound-

aries, recognizing that she could not take responsibility for her parents' choices. She could, however, take responsibility for her own: and she ended her unhealthy relationship. She started going to therapy, and reprogrammed the lies she was telling herself (that she was responsible for her family) with the truth (that she could not possibly be responsible for something over which she had no control). She began to meditate, and practice daily gratitude.

Guess what? The hair loss stopped, and regrowth began. Plus, Rachel was a lot happier.

If you think that you have stress-related hair loss, take some time to actively care for yourself and release the stress. You *can* help yourself to relax and allow your body to start healing itself.

Detox From Stress

Start by getting enough sleep. Not only will this lower your subjective experience of stress, but it has a host of other physiologic benefits.

Remember to eat a healthy diet. High sugar, high saturated fat, and nutrient deficiencies can all cause inflammation and a physiologic stress response in your body. (Additionally, if you're experiencing hair loss, it's important to ensure that you are consuming adequate calories, and adequate protein, as hair is made of protein and requires iron.)

If you are physically able, exercise regularly. Exercise elevates your mood by releasing endorphins (the natural "high") and improves your metabolism. It also promotes the elimination of toxins from your body by improving your circulation. Toxic accumulation can also cause a physiologic stress response.

Develop the ability to shift your focus. Use prayer, guided imagery, deep breathing, massage, and positive attitudes to help bring your gaze away from your problems. Revisit Chapter 9 for more on this topic!

Finally, remember to use effective communication skills and efficiency-boosting time management skills to reduce the number of things that cause you stress. With the extra time that you gain, pursue the leisure activities that put a smile on your face.

CHAPTER 17

Obstacle to Cure #8: Prolonged Poor Treatment —> Hormones Gone Haywire

The natural result of toxic living, bodily dysfunction, stress, and exhaustion is unbalanced hormones. Hormonal problems are frequently the symptom that will finally send a patient to the doctor after they have ignored all the other warning signs.

Because hormonal problems can be tricky to deal with, let's cover exactly what causes them, the conditions they create and how to test for them, and, most importantly, what to do about it.

Hypothyroidism

Your pituitary produces the hormone TSH (Thyroid Stimulating Hormone). It tells your thyroid (a gland that sits in front of your neck, right below your voice box) to produce the mostly inactive thyroid hormone T4 (so called because it has four iodine atoms bound to it). T4 then travels to your peripheral tissues, where it gets converted to T3 (meaning it loses one iodine), and becomes active. The active hormone T3 is heavily involved in controlling your metabolism.

Tyrosine, iodine, selenium, zinc and a number of other necessary nutritional cofactors are used as building blocks to create active thyroid hormone. This is more likely the cause of hypothyroidism if the diet is especially poor, or there's some other malabsorption syndrome present.

Hashimoto's, or antibodies against the thyroid, is a very common cause of hypothyroidism. Autoimmunity in general has its own set of causality, usually leading back to the gut (see Chapter 15). However, production of thyroid hormone creates oxidative stress, which requires selenium for clean-up. Without this clean-up, autoimmunity can set in. So selenium deficiency may be one risk factor.

Hypothyroidism can also be caused by mercury toxicity. Heavy metals in general are bad news, but mercury particularly can antagonize selenium, which, as has been mentioned, is necessary for multiple steps of thyroid hormone production.

It is also possible to unintentionally suppress thyroid activity with prescription drugs. Amiodarone and lithium are two well-documented examples of thyroid suppressing drugs.

The tests for hypothyroidism are easy, but the interpretation is often far from straightforward. Most doctors will run labs for TSH only, or occasionally T4. Elevated TSH means that the thyroid isn't responding to the signal from the pituitary, so the pituitary effectively "shouts louder." Sometimes, though, the thyroid remains unresponsive. It is possible for TSH and total T4 to both be normal, while patients are still functionally hypothyroid.

Functional hypothyroidism can be caused by higher circulating TBG (thyroxine-binding globulin). T4 and T3 hormones that are bound to TBG are not available to stimulate receptors. This is a good reason to test free T4 and free T3, not just the total amounts of both. One possible cause for high TBG is estrogen dominance, which can also cause a host of female hormonal problems... more on this in a bit![4]

A sluggish liver can also cause hypothyroidism. About 60% of your T4 gets converted to T3 in your liver... a process requiring selenium (again) and magnesium. If your liver is backed up (and one way to tell is if you have had a history of toxic exposure, and if you are chemically sensitive now), this might not happen efficiently.

Functional hypothyroidism is sometimes also hidden because of a higher conversion of T4 to rT3 (reverse T3, which is inactive), instead of active T3. Your liver converts some T4 to rT3 when it has too much of the former, which, in the correct ratios, is a normal process. However, in times of high stress (read: high circulating cortisol), your body is in crisis mode. This means it needs to conserve energy to deal with the stressor, so things like growth and metabolism become a lot less important. If you're chronically stressed out all the time, this process might be ongoing.

I mention functional hypothyroidism because many patients that have normal lab results have classic hypothyroid symptoms which are relieved by thyroid support or supplementation. Some symptoms to watch out for are sensitivity to cold, difficulty concentrating, constipation,
depression, fatigue (and possibly weakness), heavy menstrual bleeding, joint/muscle pain, thinning eyebrows, brittle hair or fingernails, and unintentional weight gain.

You can support your thyroid by drinking filtered water, minimizing bread products, taking a high quality multivitamin and fish oil, buying wild-caught

Pacific seafood, and minimizing stress. If you don't have adequate selenium in your diet, four brazil nuts daily will give you your daily dose—or you can supplement with no more than 200 mcg daily. And, if you think that your sluggish thyroid is caused by toxicity, try a liver cleanse and consider having your mercury amalgams replaced (by a holistic dentist who knows what he or she is doing!)

If thyroid medication is required, I prefer to treat hypothyroidism with NatureThroid or Armour (glandular products containing T1, T2, T3, T4, and calcitonin, as well as the building blocks to repair the thyroid), since in my experience, patients do much better on those than on Synthroid (T4 only).

Halides and Your Hormones

Halides (bromine and fluoride) are one of the classes of compounds that adversely affect our endocrine signaling system, and are one possible cause of the epidemic of hypothyroidism.

Bromine is an antibacterial agent used in pools and hot tubs, an agricultural fumigant, and a fumigant for pests and termites. It is in brominated vegetable oils found in sodas and beverages, and it's still in some medications, particularly for asthma.

But probably most significantly, bromine is

added to bread and bakery products as an anti-caking agent. Back in the 1960s, iodine was added to baking products instead of bromine for the same purpose. But because the therapeutic window for iodine is low, there was concern that this would disrupt thyroid function. Therefore it was replaced with bromine in the 1980s, and bromine continues to be used to this day.

Fluorine is found in the water supply in many areas, as well as in toothpastes. Most of us know (or think we know) that fluoride reduces the incidence of cavities; however, studies now suggest that fluoridation of the water makes no difference in rates of cavities.[1]

Another halide, iodine, is a critical nutrient for thyroid function. But because of the chemical similarity between iodine and its cousins bromine and fluorine, the latter two can mimic iodine in the body, binding to its receptors. These other halides block the body's uptake of iodine, potentially leading to goiter and hypothyroidism.[2]

There is a test available through specialty labs that shows urinary excretion levels of fluorine, bromine, and iodine. This can indicate how big a problem these halides may be for you. You can limit your exposure to halides in the following ways:

- **Eating organic food.** Crops that have been fumigated are likely to have elevated levels of bromine.[3]

- **Limit bakery products.** If you eat bread, make your own! Manufacturers are not required to list potassium bromate or brominated flour on the label. Or, my favorite bromine-free store-bought brand is sprouted, 100% whole grain Ezekiel bread.

- **Get a multivitamin that contains iodine**, and/or consume seaweed, unless you have Hashimoto's Thyroiditis, in which case you will want to limit your iodine intake until your antibodies are negative (as iodine can worsen the disease). Iodine and other halides are at odds with one another, and supplementing with one can supplant the other.

- **Properly salt your food.** There is good salt and bad salt, as mentioned in Chapter 2; what you want is the iodized Celtic Sea Salt, added to taste, and not the highly manufactured high-sodium containing foods. But it's not just the iodine that will help supplant fluoride and bromide—it's also the chloride, as chloride is also in the halide family. For this reason, a low-salt diet is likely to exacerbate halide toxicity.

- Avoid fluoride and fluorine by **filtering your water** and **choosing a fluoride-free toothpaste.** Filtering your water will also reduce your exposure to chlorine, which is a highly carcinogenic halogen.

The Iodine/Hormone Connection

Iodine is one of the key nutrients required for the formation of thyroid hormone, and for that reason, the thyroid requires more iodine than any other tissue in the body. Sufficient iodine intake is critically important for multiple hormonal pathways, but the body prioritizes the production of thyroid hormones when there is limited iodine intake.

Because it needs it, it takes it: the thyroid "traps" iodine first, before any other tissue can get it. But if there's not enough iodine to go around, the thyroid will swell up to try to trap it more efficiently. This is called a goiter, and it used to be really common, before iodine was added to salt in parts of the country too far away from the sea to have much iodine in the soil. But there are other tissues that require a lot of iodine: the breasts, the ovaries, and the prostate.

To understand the connection between iodine, the breasts, and the ovaries, it is necessary to first discuss the different types of estrogen. The three main types of estrogen are Estrone (called E1), Estradiol (called E2), and Estriol (called E3).

Estrone is found in fat cells, and can convert into estradiol or estriol. Estradiol is the strongest of the estrogens, and responsible for most of what we think of as "estrogenic" symptoms, both in PMS and in menopause. Under the wrong conditions, it can be metabolized into 16-Hydroxyestrogen (16-OH), which is carcinogenic (cancer-forming).

Estriol, however, has been shown to protect against estrogenic cancers, decreases the risk of fibrocystic changes in the breasts, and can even help women with estrogen-related weight changes to drop the extra pounds.

Why this is relevant: iodine helps to maintain the estrogen balance in favor of estriol.

(There are other ways to increase estriol, too, by the way: one great one is to increase your intake of cruciferous veggies such as broccoli, cauliflower, cabbage, and brussels sprouts, due to their high concentration of Di-indole-methane (DIM). Just make sure you wilt them first, or they may block uptake of iodine. Then you'll be working at cross purposes!)

But alas: iodine is a common nutritional deficiency not only because it is blocked by halides, but also because it is hard to find in food. It exists only in low concentrations in the soil. To some extent this is natural (as you get farther away from the ocean), but it is also partially due to farming practices that deplete the soil of many nutrients, of which iodine is one.

Also, the iodine added to table salt is generally a

reduced form called iodide. Iodide works just fine for the thyroid, but not for the breasts, ovaries, or prostate. (And again, table salt isn't the healthiest choice of salt for you anyway, as mentioned in Chapter 2).

As I mentioned, the best way to get iodine is from seaweed or a multivitamin. Not everybody needs iodine though, so get your levels checked before you start supplementing with large doses of it (what's in your multivitamin is probably fine). Also, again, get checked for antibodies against your thyroid, as iodine can make Hashimoto's worse if it is present.

Nina, 33, came to me after a self-breast exam revealed a lump that had not been present before. She was understandably concerned, though she did tell me that the day before, she'd suffered some blunt trauma to the breast in question, in the exact spot where she now found the lesion. We sent her for an ultrasound just to be sure, and found that it was indeed a simple cyst, most likely secondary to the trauma. The radiologist told her that sometimes cysts disappear on their own, and sometimes they get bigger, but as long as it wasn't bothering her, she might as well leave it alone.

On her own, Nina (who fortunately did not have Hashimoto's) started taking 12.5 mg of iodine daily, due to some subclinical hypothyroid symptoms such as occasional constipation and cold extremities. While those symptoms did not go away, she did report that afterwards, her periods became much lighter, her premenstrual breast tenderness went away—and the breast cyst vanished within a month!

Acne and Your Thyroid

Common causes of acne include hormone imbalance, a backed up liver, elevated androgens (hormones in the testosterone family) sometimes due to PCOS, too-high sugar and insulin resistance, and occasionally low essential fatty acids. But sometimes, acne can be a symptom of hypothyroidism. Here's why.

One common correlate to hypothyroidism is elevated cholesterol. This is because when thyroid levels are low, the liver isn't filtering the cholesterol out of the bloodstream as quickly as it should—which means it won't be available to the body tissues that need cholesterol to form all the stuff cholesterol makes. The most important of these in this case is progesterone.

Why this is important? Progesterone facilitates the release of thyroid hormone from the thyroid gland, while estrogen blocks it (which is why estrogen dominance and hypothyroidism tend to coexist).

Adequate Vitamin A is also necessary for the formation of progesterone... but there's another reason why Vitamin A is important.

The best known treatment for acne involves retinoid drugs, which are derivatives of Vitamin A. Vitamin A works by encouraging the regeneration of keratin in the skin (which is why it's also in most anti-aging formulas).Vitamin A is a fat-soluble vitamin, found in liver, meat, eggs, and dairy. Its water-soluble precursor, carotenoids, are found in red, yellow, and orange veggies.

However, if your thyroid is sluggish, you won't be able to effectively convert carotenoids to Vitamin A, no matter how many carrots you eat. (And there's a feedback loop between the two: if you're low on Vitamin A, you won't be able to effectively convert T4 into the more active T3.)

You might have noticed that it's all interconnected: low thyroid function can cause acne. But so can a low-fat diet, since you'll be low in Vitamin A, and so can estrogen dominance (and low progesterone). But then low progesterone and low Vitamin A can also exacerbate hypothyroidism, too. The best approach to keep all these factors in balance? Balance your hormones, skip the low fat diets, and balance your thyroid.

Ashley, 25, came to me with severe cystic acne that was poorly responsive to traditional acne treatments, and joint and muscle pain. She'd tried just about everything.
After some testing, we discovered that Ashley had

Hashimoto's (antibodies against her thyroid), as well as pretty severe hypothyroidism—though her presentation was irregular, since she had none of the classic symptoms of hypothyroidism. We put her on NatureThroid, and also removed gluten and dairy from her diet, since she opted not to do food allergy testing and gluten and dairy are some of the most common culprits in Hashimoto's patients. The joint and muscle pain vanished within a few weeks of Ashley's diet change, and her skin began to improve immediately. It took us a few months to find the right   NatureThroid dose, but once we did, her skin cleared up completely.

Do be aware that while Vitamin A in high doses does treat acne, it's not a good idea to take high doses of it without supervision, as it is a fat-soluble vitamin and therefore possible to overdose. Vitamin A in high doses is also unsafe in pregnancy and should be avoided. (Balanced thyroid and progesterone hormones and sufficient dietary fat, on the other hand, are all very good ideas in pregnancy!)

"Bound" vs "Free" Hormones

When balancing your thyroid (and sex hormones), it is necessary to consider the ratio of bound hormones to free hormones.

Think of hormones as keys, and the hormone receptors as locks. When the key fits into the right doorknob, the door will open. But you don't always want the door to open—or at least you don't want too many doors to open all at the same time. The way your body gets around this is to put "sheaths" on most of the keys; that way, even if they come in contact with the right doorknob, they won't fit. The sheath is called a *binding globulin.*

Different binding globulins are specific to different hormones. The Sex Hormone Binding Globulin (SHBG) binds androgens like testosterone, DHEA, and dihydrotestosterone, as well as estrogen. The Thyroid Binding Globulin (TBG) binds thyroid. The Corticosteroid Binding Globulin (CBG) binds progesterone, cortisol, and other corticosteroids.

Binding globulins matter because **only those hormones that are not "sheathed" by a binding globulin are what we call** *bioavailable*: i.e. available to stimulate the receptors (unlock the doors).

This is why it's important to check free T3 and free T4 in a thyroid panel, not merely T3 and T4. It makes a difference how much hormone is actually unbound and bioavailable. This is also an important distinction for testosterone, since SHBG has a very high affinity for testosterone. A man can technically have a normal total testosterone level, but a low free testosterone level, which will still leave him with symptoms of low testosterone.

Bound hormones go up and down for a number

of reasons. SHBG decreases when androgens are high, such as testosterone and DHEA. This can happen from supplementation, or from conditions that cause them to spike, such as Polycystic Ovarian Syndrome (PCOS).

Hypothyroidism decreases SHBG as well, which may partially explain the correlation between hypothyroidism and other hormonal issues, such as PMS and menopausal symptoms. By the same token, high estrogen levels can increase the Thyroid Binding Globulin, leading to symptoms of hypothyroidism as well.

Obesity and excess insulin trigger lower SHBG, and low SHBG also seems to increase the incidence of diabetes. This is partly why losing weight, minimizing sugar and increasing exercise is so effective at hormone balancing: as you lose weight, SHBG goes up. Conversely, very thin or anorexic women often do not get their periods anymore, possibly due to elevated SHBG.

You can test SHBG and TBG directly, and in some cases this is clinically useful. But the first step is to test the free, unbound forms of thyroid (T3 and T4). And of the sex hormones, it is especially helpful to test the free and total levels of testosterone in men.

Women with estrogen dominance symptoms or PCOS, on the other hand, would do well to increase

SHBG with diet and lifestyle modifications: specifically, exercise more and consume two tablespoons of ground flax seeds daily!

DHEA

DHEA (Dehydroepiandrosterone) is one of three major cholesterol-based hormones produced by your adrenal glands, along with aldosterone and cortisol. DHEA is a precursor hormone for estrogen and testosterone in both men and women.

Aside from its role as a parent hormone, DHEA also counters the effects of too-high cortisol. While enough cortisol is necessary to maintain your energy and to counterbalance adrenaline, too much is a problem.

• High cortisol encourages weight gain and metabolic syndrome by increasing blood sugar and inhibiting conversion of inactive to active thyroid hormone. Conversely, DHEA encourages a faster metabolism.

• While cortisol suppresses the immune system (and inflammation), DHEA supports it. It can be very helpful in modulating autoimmunity and allergies.

• While cortisol "breaks down," thinning the skin, breaking down bones and speeding aging, DHEA "builds up," protecting against these deleterious effects. For these reasons, DHEA has been considered an anti-aging hormone.

DHEA deficiencies happen, though, because in a competition against DHEA, cortisol wins. Again, of the adrenal hormones, cortisol is the most important. Too much is a problem, but too little is disaster. If the body has to choose which to make, it'll pick cortisol every time.

As we age, this happens naturally; in our 70s we only produce about 5% as much DHEA as we produced at twenty. This may partly explain why one hallmark of aging involves using up the body's resources without building them back up again.

You may also favor cortisol, leading to a deficiency in DHEA, if you're in adrenal fatigue. Because DHEA is the parent hormone for estrogen and testosterone, sufficient quantities are necessary for hormone balancing. This is one reason why women who have adrenal fatigue have such a hard time both with PMS and in menopause.

Because DHEA is a natural substance, it is unregulated by the FDA. It's available over the counter, but be careful with taking any hormones without having your levels checked first. For women, too much DHEA typically results in an overabundance of testosterone, which can lead to abnormal hair growth, acne, and irritability. It's also possible for DHEA to convert primarily to estrogen in some women, leading to estrogen dominance symptoms such as mood swings, water retention, and breast tenderness. Men who take more DHEA than necessary will most likely find that most of it converts to estrogen.

It's important to know where your DHEA is at to begin with, and to dose only as much as you need.

PCOS (Polycystic Ovarian Syndrome)

Polycystic Ovarian Syndrome (literally, multiple ovarian cysts) presents with a few key signs and symptoms, though not all of them are present in every case.

Classically, being overweight is part of the picture, though about half of the women who have PCOS are not overweight. When patients are overweight, however, the syndrome is also associated with elevated blood sugar, insulin resistance (and downstream hypertension), or even Type 2 Diabetes.

Because of their problems with elevated androgens (testosterone, etc.), women suffering from PCOS often have irregular menstrual periods and anovulatory cycles. Anovulation, of course, causes infertility, which is another hallmark symptom of PCOS. The androgens may also cause hirsuitism (abnormal hair growth) and acne.

Because PCOS is found both in heavier and in very thin women, there may be multiple causes of the syndrome. However, estrogen dominance is always a problem in these women, often due to toxic exposures to endocrine disrupting chemicals such as phthalates, Bisphenol A, cadmium, and mercury. Arguably, insulin resistance may also be a cause, as too much insulin decreases Sex Hormone Binding Globulin (SHBG), which leads to more circulating androgens.

Women diagnosed with PCOS tend to have labs that show an elevated ratio of LH:FSH (the hormones in your brain that tell your ovaries to produce estrogen), too-high androgens (usually testosterone, free and total, as well as DHEA, leading to acne and hirsuitism and suppressing ovulation). Insulin is also sometimes (but not always) elevated, and cholesterol can be elevated as well, as part of the metabolic syndrome picture.

Diagnosis is a combination of symptoms, biochemical signs (those that show up on the labs), and imaging (an ultrasound showing multiple ovarian cysts), combined with exclusion of other possible causes.

Some of the classical treatment options for PCOS include Metformin (a diabetes medication, for those women whose PCOS symptoms include metabolic syndrome) and birth control (to regulate LH:FSH production and suppress over-production of androgens).

From a naturopathic standpoint, the treatment will look somewhat different depending on the woman's symptoms (for example, if she doesn't have metabolic syndrome then we won't be focusing on regulating blood sugar, and if she's clearly had a toxic exposure to endocrine-disrupting chemicals, then detox will be a big part of the protocol). But one treatment I almost always include is inositol.

Inositol is present in muscle tissue as myoinositol. Inositol regulates both FSH and TSH (thyroid stimulating hormone), and also plays a role in regulating insulin levels. I consider it to be an outstanding treatment based on some very impressive studies: In one study, women who received inositol versus those who received placebo demonstrated a higher ovulation rate (25% compared to 15%) and a shorter time to first ovulation (24.5 days compared to 40.5 days).[5] In another study, women in the group receiving inositol saw a significant decrease in serum testosterone (both free and total), plasma triglycerides, blood pressure, and insulin levels.[6] And in yet another study, researchers compared Metformin treatment with inositol, showing a significant increase in ovulation (65% compared to 50%) and in pregnancy (30% compared to 18.3%) in the group re-ceiving inositol.[7]

Kelly, 29, came to me initially with severe acne. Her lab work confirmed that her testosterone levels were very high and her LH:FSH ratio was almost 4:1. She also craved sweets and ate mostly fast food, and suffered with gas and bloating characteristic of candida overgrowth. Over a period of months, we slowly improved her diet un-til she was able to tolerate the candida protocol, while putting her on quite a few hormone balancing herbs, as well as inositol.

About six months later, Kelly's skin was clear and her gut healthy. She decided she was ready to try to get preg-nant, and so I taught her how to chart her cycles to deter-mine whether she was ovulating or not, and also sent her for more lab work to determine where her LH:FSH ratio was now. When she sent me her charts, I was perplexed to see that she still was not ovulating. When she came for her next appointment, though, I found out that was be-cause she was already pregnant!

The bottom line is that combined with appropri-ate protocols to address blood sugar, cholesterol, in-sulin levels, hypertension, and clinical symptoms of high androgens, there are definitely good treatment options out there for PCOS. Inositol is high on my list—in combination with a full protocol to balance estrogen dominance.

PMS & Cramping

PMS is usually correlated with a high ratio of estrogen to progesterone. Although both hormones decline dramatically leading up to your period, if you have relatively more circulating estrogen than progesterone, you're probably going to have an unpleasant week or so.

Most of us associate PMS with mood swings and cramping, but many other symptoms such as insomnia, poor concentration, joint or muscle pain, fatigue, headaches and migraines, bloating, acne (especially around the chin and neck for many women), changing bowel habits, water retention and weight gain may be related.

Traditional Treatments

Many doctors will prescribe synthetic hormone-based birth control pills in an effort to treat PMS and regulate your cycle. These are often effective, and while many women do fine on them, there are some long-term consequences which you should keep in mind, such as increased risk of certain cancers and of stroke (especially for women over 35 who smoke). The Pill itself may also cause imbalance in gut flora, mood swings, acne, weight gain, decreased libido, and fertility problems later on (as mentioned in

Chapter 12).

If your PMS symptoms are mild, you may be able to control the cramping and muscle pain quite well with over the counter anti-inflammatory medications such as Advil or ibuprofen. Although these too have their side effects with continued long-term use, once in awhile I see no problem with them for most patients, aside from the fact that they don't address the reason the pain is there in the first place.

For water retention, your doctor may give you diuretics (to make you urinate more). They work, but again, they don't deal with the reason you're retaining water in the first place.

For severe PMS, you may be given antidepressants, which help not just with stabilizing mood, but also have been effective for reducing some of the other symptoms as well. Common side effects for these include GI disturbance, sexual side effects such as lowered libido, insomnia, and occasionally they can actually intensify feelings of depression (see Chapter 12).

Naturopathic PMS Treatments

As with most conditions, it's important to start with what you eat. I recommend a high fiber (fruits and veggies), low sugar, and low refined carbohydrate diet, as this helps to restore the balance of gut flora and increase SHBG.

Exercise is also very important: studies show that women who exercise experience significantly fewer PMS symptoms. This is also likely due to the increase in SHBG.

High estrogen levels can increase the Thyroid Binding Globulin, decreasing the bioavailable thyroid hormone. By the same token, hypothyroidism can decrease SHBG, contributing to estrogen dominance. But regardless of which came first, if you have PMS and any thyroid issues, both will need to be addressed for either one to truly improve.

I also recommend liver and gut support, probably at the same time. You may have high levels of estrogen because "bad" bacteria in your gut keeps it from getting eliminated, or because a backed up liver can't do its job properly, or a combination of both. At the very least, I'd recommend a high quality probiotic of at least 20 billion organisms, with a 50/50 ratio of bifidobacillus to lactobacillus. Topical castor oil packs are also a great idea to assist with liver detox.

To create a castor oil pack, you will need cold pressed castor oil and a flannel sheet. Fold the flannel sheet to about the size of your liver, underneath the right side of your rib cage, and saturate one side of it with castor oil. Apply over your liver, and wrap seran wrap around your body to keep it in place. Place a heating pad on top, and relax for about 30-45 minutes. The castor oil penetrates the skin well, causing a local "inflammatory" reaction (in a good way), telling your body, "Hey, there's something to pay attention to here!" This will draw more blood flow to your liver, which means more oxygen, more nutrients, and faster waste elimination—causing your liver to "dump" into your colon. It's a good way to facilitate the liver's normal physiologic function, but a little faster and more efficiently than usual.

Make sure you're on a good fish oil in order to decrease inflammation, as omega 3 fatty acids function much like ibuprofen but without the side effects. As mentioned in Chapter 2, shoot for about 1 gram daily of EPA.

Magnesium can also help to relieve cramping or lower back pain.

There are also a number of botanical medications which work wonders for hormone balancing—one of my favorites is Chaste Tree, also known as Vitex.

Sometimes I prescribe progesterone for PMS and cramping. Most of the time this isn't necessary, but it will get the job done, and with far fewer side effects than those encountered with birth control pills.

Bioidentical Hormone Replacement Therapy (BHRT)

Estrogen has receptors in just about every part of a woman's body and contributes to health of the urinary tract, bones and muscles, blood vessels, skin and vaginal tissue. But, there can be too much of a good thing: once again, estrogen dominance (relative to progesterone) leads to symptoms like PMS, mood swings, cramping, fluid retention, fibroids and heavy bleeding, low libido, elevated cholesterol and triglycerides.

Progesterone helps to prepare the uterine lining for implantation, and so it begins to rise just after ovulation. Progesterone and estrogen decline together throughout the second half of a woman's menstrual cycle, and if the two are in balance, the symptoms associated with estrogen dominance should not occur.

Women also produce testosterone—about 1/20 of the amount of testosterone that men produce. Testosterone contributes to healthy libido, a sense of well-being and vitality, and healthy bones and muscles. When a woman is estrogen dominant, she may be clinically deficient in testosterone even if her blood levels of total testosterone are normal, since too much estrogen produces Sex Hormone Binding Globulin (SHBG). This protein binds testosterone, rendering it unavailable to the cells for use. (Again, that's why it's useful to check not just total testosterone on blood tests, but free testosterone. This gives you a more complete clinical picture.)

Until July 2002, Premarin, Progestins, and

Methyltestosterone were the standard estrogen, progesterone, and testosterone replacement treatments for
menopausal symptoms. However, the Heart and Es-
trogen/progestin Replacement Study (HERS) and
Women's Health Initiative (WHI) clinical trials illu-
minated the health risks associated with synthetic
hormones. Bioidentical hormones, however, were not
included in these trials, and do not carry the same
risks.

Premarin is an estrogen replacement drug prepared from pregnant horse urine. These are conjugat-
ed estrogens, and they are not biologically identical
to those produced in the body—which means they do
not follow normal human metabolic pathways. They
are associated with vaginal bleeding, high blood
pressure, blood clots, stroke, heart disease, nausea,
vomiting, headaches, fluid retention, and they may
increase the risk of estrogen receptor positive
cancers.

Progestins are synthetic progesterone molecules,
are less effective than bioidentical progesterone, and
can cause side effects such as abnormal menses or
loss of menses, nausea, depression, weight changes,
fluid retention, and insomnia.

Methyltestosterone is a synthetic analog of testosterone that puts added stress on the liver, and is correlated with liver damage and liver cancer. The body

does not recognize it, so it is not possible to correlate clinical effects of methyltestosterone with blood levels of testosterone.

Bioidentical hormones are still prepared in a lab, but the molecules themselves are identical to those produced in the body (hence the name). Prescriptions will depend upon the individual's levels of each of the hormones, as well as her symptoms.

Bioidentical progesterone is prepared from extracts of wild yam or soybeans. Progesterone counterbalances estrogen dominance symptoms, helps lift mood, restores libido (by counterbalancing estrogen), improves memory, assists with sleep, and protects against endometrial cancer. It may, however, alter the timing of the menstrual cycle for women who are still menstruating.

Unlike methyltestosterone, it is possible to correlate blood levels with clinical activity for bioidentical testosterone. I usually prescribe this only when both the symptoms and blood levels agree. Since testosterone is a controlled substance, women whose prescription includes testosterone must have blood levels checked every six months, as opposed to yearly for just estrogen and progesterone. It is possible to overdose on testosterone—symptoms of overdose include aggression and irritability, acne, and abnormal hair growth.

* * *

Candice felt like she was crawling out of her skin. She'd had her last period over a year before the first time I saw her, and had a few hot flashes and night sweats since. But it wasn't until her work schedule forced her to commute from Tucson to Phoenix on a daily basis to oversee the development of a new wing of her company that she really began to suffer. After that, Candice had multiple hot flashes per day, and woke up each night soaked in sweat. Her "fuse," or stress tolerance, was almost zero: she was excessively irritable, snapping at her husband at the slightest provocation (even when she knew it wasn't his fault!)

At the next follow up visit, Candice was a new person. While her work schedule had not yet calmed down, she was much better equipped to tolerate the stress. Hot flashes and night sweats were gone, she slept through the night, and her mood had evened out.

How to (Naturally) Increase Testosterone Levels

Women are not the only ones that can have problems with low testosterone. As men age, testosterone levels naturally decline. There are several reasons for this, but one of them is an increase in SHBG (Sex Hormone Binding Globulin). Again, this binds testosterone and keeps it from actively stimulating receptors.

Another reason involves the obesity epidemic. (Men, if you need still more motivation to lose weight, here it is!) Your fat cells (adipose tissue) contain an enzyme called aromitase. Aromitase converts testosterone into its sister steroid hormone: estrogen. Not only does having a beer belly lower testosterone levels, then; it actually increases estrogen levels at the same time (which can also cause breast tissue to develop in men—gynecomastia.)

But these days, it's not uncommon for even younger men to have low testosterone levels. Controlling for age and other factors, testosterone levels have declined across the population over the past two decades by about 20%. This means that a 50 year old man now will have 20% less testosterone than a similarly healthy 50 year old did in 1993.[8]

There has been much speculation regarding the cause of this decline. One of them involves environmental toxins. Many commonly used chemicals have an endocrine-disrupting effect (i.e. they screw up your hormones), including phthalates, parabens, diethanolamine, triethanolamine, monoethanolamine, and toluene, to name a few.

Another possibility is the obsession with lowering cholesterol. Testosterone is a cholesterol-based hormone; you must have sufficient cholesterol in order to make it. Conventional wisdom tells us to avoid cholesterol, and very common cholesterol-lowering drugs (statins) stop the liver from producing cholesterol altogether, which means that everything down-stream doesn't get produced either. This includes bile salts (which help us digest fat—where we also get our fat soluble vitamins), vitamin D, healthy cell membranes (vital for your health, as mentioned in Chapter 2), and steroid hormones (such as testos-terone, estrogen, progesterone, and DHEA, among others). An estimated 32 million Americans are on statins, so this could certainly account for part of the testosterone decline.

There's also a great deal of debate surrounding phytoestrogens, such as soy. While there are numer-ous health benefits from the isoflavones in soy, prob-ably everyone (not just men) should avoid GMO soy —which most of it is—just to be on the safe side.

The two most commonly known effects of testos-terone are sexual virility and increased muscle mass, so this means that lower testosterone can also lead to sexual dysfunction and/or lowered muscle mass (with a corresponding increase in body fat). But low testos-terone can also manifest as depression, low bone mineral density, low energy, and anemia.

To make enough testosterone, you need to get enough sleep. Sleep helps you lose weight, decreases your stress levels, and increases the secretion of testosterone as well as Growth Hormone, both of which help to build and repair muscle mass.

It is also helpful to lose weight. Losing weight does not mean eating a low fat diet, but a low sugar diet. As a cholesterol-based hormone, eating animal products (where cholesterol is found) actually boosts your testosterone levels. (Perhaps there's a reason why men stereotypically love steak! The caveat to this, though: make sure you're eating clean, grass-fed meat when at all possible. And increase your intake of healthy fats.)

In general, don't eat processed crap full of chemicals. Your liver has several jobs, but the most important is to detoxify foreign chemicals. If your liver is busy detoxing, it won't be able to perform its other jobs effectively, such as breaking down complex molecules (like estrogen) so they can be eliminated from your body, or breaking down fat (where aromitase is stored, converting testosterone to estrogen). It's also important to eat your serving of veggies, especially cruciferous veggies, as these are great for helping your liver perform more efficiently.

Nicotine and other additives in cigarettes actually decrease testosterone production.[9] That means you need to stop smoking!

Exercise can raise testosterone levels. Cardio is good, but resistance training (to build muscle) is better; training large muscles like your quadriceps and hamstrings is best of all for boosting testosterone. If you're already in pretty good shape, you should focus on muscle building (as opposed to toning), which involves higher weight and lower repetitions. If you're not already in good shape, start where you are and go from there.

Another helpful tip: chill out. Stress (particularly feeling trapped or helpless) decreases your testosterone levels. Pick a few stress management techniques that appeal to you, and give them a try.

And, to protect yourself from too many estrogens, avoid toxins—especially those in your toiletry items.

How Caffeine Affects Your Hormones

I'll be honest: I love coffee. Coffee consumption in moderation decreases the risk of many chronic diseases. But especially if you're a woman with estrogen dominance issues or low libido, mounting evidence suggests that coffee consumption in excess of two cups per day may make it worse.

All foreign chemicals have to go through either your liver or your kidneys to get broken down into simple enough pieces to get eliminated. Your liver has lots of different "queues" (called cytochrome systems) for breaking stuff down. Each chemical has to go through its own particular queue before it can get out of the body. And, as we all know, the longer the line, the longer it takes to check out.

It just so happens that caffeine and estrogen share the same cytochrome system (CYP1A2).

The logical conclusion here is that excessive coffee consumption worsens estrogen dominance, because while your liver is dealing with caffeine, estrogen can't get eliminated fast enough at that proper time of the month... making PMS, cramping, acne, fibrocystic breasts and any number of menstrual-related symptoms worse.

Holly, 23, was basically healthy but came to me because she'd noticed lumps in her breasts and was concerned about them. We did a breast exam, and discovered not a discrete lump, but many ropy fibrocystic changes. I asked her how much coffee she drank daily, and she told me she pretty much drank it all day long!

I told her that while I was happy to send her for an ultrasound to put her mind at ease, I strongly suspected that some diet and lifestyle changes were all that was needed to reverse the problem. We put her on a diet protocol consisting primarily of whole foods, tapered her down to a reasonable 12 oz cup per day of coffee, and gave her a multivitamin and fish oil.

Sure enough, within a few cycles her breasts were healthy and normal.

As a matter of fact, a research study found that more than 100 mg of caffeine daily (a normal cup of coffee contains 95-200 mg) will increase circulating estrogen levels to some degree, but up to 500 mg daily (around 4-5 cups) will increase circulating estrogen levels by 70%![10]

Excessive coffee consumption does not just impact women though. As both men and women grow older, production of testosterone correspondingly declines. For men, obviously adequate testosterone levels are crucial. For women, testosterone is also important for maintaining libido, building muscle, and maintaining metabolism. But research shows that the more caffeine you consume, the lower your bioavailable testosterone levels will be.[11] This is apparently because caffeine increases Sex Hormone Binding Globulin (SHBG), which will bind testosterone and prevent it from doing you any good.

One or a max of two cups of (caffeinated) coffee daily will help you to reap the antioxidant and blood sugar support benefits of coffee… but don't go over two, or you'll risk the potential damage of abusing your adrenal glands as well as screwing up your hormones.

Recap: How to Balance Your Hormones

If your hormones are out of balance, the first step is to get a blood test (or a salivary test, as the case may be, or an ultrasound) to identify the source of the problem. Balancing will likely involve supplementation, possibly with the hormones you are lacking.

In the meantime, though, all the other "basic building blocks" in Part 2 of this book work together in concert to assist with hormone balancing. Make sure they're in place!

CHAPTER 18

Obstacle to Cure #9: Toxic Thoughts and Limiting Beliefs

As mentioned in the introductory cases, this obstacle to cure often plays a role, at least in conjunction with some of the others. We're experts at lying to ourselves, and our beliefs become our reality. Here's why.

Thoughts have a physical structure in your brain, and they can trigger emotions, which set off a cascade of hormones that cause physiologic changes in your body. If you meditate on negative things ("I'm a failure, I will never succeed, the universe is against me, I will never get well, I'm not responsible for the course of my life," etc), this will influence your words; your words will influence your choices; your choices become your actions; and your actions will determine many of your life circumstances.

The Bible often refers to the heart as the seat of emotions and also the part of us that generates thoughts and beliefs (Mark 2:8, Luke 5:22). God tells us that we are to guard our hearts "above all else", for it is the "wellspring of life" (Prov 4:23).

But how do we do that?

Recognize that thoughts are real, physical things.

Your body has to translate a thought or idea into a real thing in order for it to be stored in your brain. Brain cells, or neurons, look like trees. Thoughts and memories get stored in these neurons, and as you accumulate more information, the branches of those trees get bigger.

Fear and *anger* both trigger the fight-or flight stress hormones you learned about in Chapter 13. Short term, these lead to sweating, shortness of breath and a rapid heart rate. Over time, however, chronically elevated stress hormones can lead to high blood pressure, high cholesterol, heart disease, diabetes, insomnia, sexual dysfunction, anxiety, constipation, diarrhea, immune dysfunction, depression, and even cancer.

Depression has a number of physical side effects,

including a lower threshold for pain, chronic fatigue, decreased interest in sex, decreased appetite, and either insomnia or hypersomnia.

Anxiety, or worrying, can have effects very similar to chronic fear. Long term effects include immune suppression, digestive disturbance, tense muscles, heart disease, and memory loss, in addition to those listed under fear and anger.

This is why your thoughts deserve attention— what you think about becomes a part of your brain, and sets off a cascade of physiological effects throughout your body. There's no such thing as "just a thought"! Solomon said, "As a man thinks in his heart, so is he" (Prov 23:7).

It's also true that a thought might not set off a cascade of physically damaging hormones—but it may instead keep you stuck, and prevent you from achieving your goals. If you believe you are *not* responsible for the things that are under your control, including your needs, your desires, and feelings, then you are lying to yourself (more on this in Chapter 13). And that lie can keep you from doing what you need to do in order to get those needs, desires, and feelings met.

So the next step is to identify your specific enemy: what is the lie, and how can you recognize it?

* * *

Become aware of what you're thinking about.

Stop and listen to your internal dialogue. What are you telling yourself? What kinds of emotions are you experiencing as a result of those internal statements? If you're frustrated about a particular situation you're in, listen to how you talk to yourself about that situation.

This might take practice. Sit down in a quiet space and stay there until your mind quiets down. Then ask yourself questions in order to follow a train of thought to its root.

A few examples:

- I feel (*an emotion: anger, fear, depression, anxiety, etc*). Why? Where does this emotion come from? How long has it been there?
  - What is it that I am fearing?
  - What is it that I am upset about?
  - What is it that I am thinking?

Continue to ask yourself "why" to the responses of each of these questions until you come up with a statement that involves only you; nobody else. These are the core issues that you can take to the next step. Some examples:

- I believe that I will only be loved if I am perfect or easy to deal with.
- I believe that I will fail at everything I do.
- I believe someone else or some other entity is responsible for making my life work out the way I want it to.

Sometimes it's helpful to know where these beliefs stem from, what event in our lives allowed these lies to take root, but sometimes it isn't necessary. You will most likely know when this is or is not important. If you feel you need an answer to this question, stick with it until you get one. Don't be afraid to seek professional help to unravel these questions if you need to—that's what counselors are there for!

Now, for the next step: the Bible tells us that we are to "demolish arguments and every pretension that sets itself up against the knowledge of God, and *we take captive every thought* to make it obedient to Christ" (2 Cor 10:5). This means we are *not* powerless to control the thoughts we think. *We are in control of what we think about.* Like wild animals, running through our yard, we can cage up our thoughts.

Accept or Reject Your Thoughts

Decide which thoughts to accept and which to reject based on whether they are 1) truth or a lie, and 2) helpful or harmful to you.

I make this distinction, because even a true thought may not be worth the real estate in your mind, if it is not "honorable, right, pure, lovely, of good repute, excellent, or worthy of praise," as Paul says in Philippians 4:8. Choose to accept only those thoughts that meet *both* criteria.

This is a conscious decision. When you identify a thought as being either a lie or harmful to your well-being, rebuke it and break its authority over your life, out loud. Refuse to accept it. Thoughts become words; that's why Jesus said, "Out of the abundance of the heart, the mouth speaks" (Matt 12:34). The reverse is also true; what you confess with your mouth eventually makes its way into your heart (Romans 10:9).

Once you have done this, you must *rapidly* replace the negative thought with something positive (and true)—otherwise, you will eventually be overcome, and "the final condition of that man is worse than the first" (Matt 12:45).

Reprogram the toxic thought with the truth.

The Bible says: "Do not conform any longer to the pattern of this world, but be transformed by the renewing of your mind. Then you will be able to test and approve what God's will is—his good, pleasing, and perfect will" (Romans 12:2).

You renew your mind with the Word of God (Eph 6:17; 2 Tim 3:16). This means you must find the specific promises to counteract the particular lie you are believing, and speak them out loud!

- If you lack confidence, find the verses that tell you your identity in Christ.
- If you believe you are not loved, find the verses that say you are.
- If you believe you are being cheated or slighted, find verses that promise justice.
- If you struggle with finances, find verses that promise provision.
- If you struggle with illness, find verses that promise health.
- If you struggle with anxiety, focus on verses that promise comfort and peace.
- If you don't know what decision to make, focus on verses that promise direction.
- If you feel the world is against you, focus on verses that promise favor.
- If you struggle with fear, focus on verses that remind you of God's faithfulness and the fact that He is worthy of trust.

- If you deal with depression, focus on verses that promise you the joy of the Lord.
- If you feel impotent, focus on verses that promise power.
- If you feel threatened, focus on verses that promise safety.
- If you feel like a failure, focus on verses that promise success and victory.

All of these verses exist in scripture, and there are a lot of them. I recommend you scour the Bible for your own promises, because the verses you find on your own will mean the most to you. You value what you "pay" for, after all—and in this case, if you put in the effort to find your own verses, you will be much more likely to put in the effort to follow the steps and reprogram your mind. (Because let's be honest—that's not easy.)

If you're not a Christian, can you still use this process to your advantage? Yes. Scriptural principles work, no matter who you are… the trick will be getting yourself to believe what you are saying, if you don't have an underlying trust that the promise came from Someone you can rely upon.

As you begin to reprogram your mind with the Word of God, your faith will grow, because "Faith comes by hearing, and hearing by the Word of

God" (Romans 10:17). But it won't happen overnight. The Word of God is like a seed (Matt 13:22-23), and seeds do not spring up immediately after they are planted. Rather, they come up "first the stalk, then the head, and then the full kernel in the head" (Mark 4:28). Because of this, realize that you will need to tell yourself the truth for some time before it begins to take root and grow. But it will bear fruit in time, and the fruits of the Spirit are the positive thoughts you want: "love, joy, peace, forbearance, kindness, goodness, faithfulness, gentleness, and self control" (Gal 5:22-23).

Every time a toxic thought encroaches in your life, repeat steps 2-4.

If it is a lie that you have already identified and rebuked, simply use the faith that you have cultivated to extinguish it (Eph 6:16). If it is a new lie, identify the lie, find the scriptures that counteract it and tell yourself the truth from the Word of God until the seed takes root in your heart, springs forth and bears fruit.

From personal experience, this works. When I first started my medical practice, with no idea how to grow a business and over $100K in debt to pay back, I had maybe two patients per week if I was lucky. It was a terrifying time. But *fortunately, I knew these principles.*

So here's what I did: I rehearsed my victories. I wrote out every time in my life that the situation looked impossible, and yet God came through. When I'd exhausted that, I wrote out every time in the lives of people I knew that the situation looked impossible, and God came through. When I ran out of those, I went through the Old Testament and found every story I could when the situation looked impossible... and God came through.

Then I wrote out every verse in my little database that promised that God is the same, yesterday, today, and forever. He will not change.

Then I wrote out only the best verses (there were too many!) listing all the specific promises above: provision, success, victory, direction, blessings upon my hard work...

Then I wrote out James 1:2-4, which says, "Count it all joy, my brothers, when you meet trials of various kinds, for you know that the testing of your faith produces steadfastness. And let steadfastness have its full effect, that you may be perfect and complete, lacking in nothing." I praised God that my trials were performing that work in me, producing steadfastness, so that in the future I would not waver in the presence of seemingly insurmountable obstacles. I would be better equipped the next time.

When this was all done, it totaled around 17 pages in my journal. Every time I caught myself beginning to panic, I pulled out my journal and reread those 17 pages, out loud. At first I had to do this almost five times per day. But eventually that went down to four times, and then three, and two, and one... and then I had it. I'd effectively reprogrammed my mind to believe and not doubt.

It wasn't quick, but I did eventually see the substance

of my faith materialize: my business grew and began to succeed, and I began to pay down my loans in record time. But even better, I'd produced a step-by-step process that I could use in the next time of trial in my own life, and I could also share it with patients as they faced struggles from which there appeared to be no way out.

Indeed, "the testing of our faith produces steadfastness," if we do not give up.

Blessings to you!

CONCLUSION

When I first started practicing naturopathic medicine, I felt intimidated by the breadth of different illnesses that might confront me. How could I possibly know how to treat every one of them? Even after medical school, even with all my references and careful study and resources, it just seemed overwhelming.

But the longer I've been in practice, the more I've come to truly trust in the simplicity of naturopathic medicine. There are only so many building blocks, and there are only so many potential obstacles to cure. Get familiar with those, and it doesn't really matter what the particular disease happens to be called—the approach is still quite similar. More often than not, the patient will lead me to the right answer if I just ask enough questions and listen well.

But you, the patient, still bear the lion's share of the work. While system imbalances usually do require intervention and guidance from a physician, after that the real work of healing depends upon you. You're the one who will have to avoid those obstacles to cure going forward, and you're the one who must create the environment in which health and healing can prevail.

I hope this guide has helped you to identify your own obstacles to cure, and begin adding in those building blocks that you are lacking. If you still need more guidance, I highly recommend that you find a licensed naturopathic physician in your area. A great resource to locate one is the American Association of Naturopathic Physicians website: just go to "Find an ND," type in your zip code, and you will see all of those located in your area. If there are none in your zip code, just broaden your search; at this point, even in states that are technically unlicensed (meaning naturopathic physicians are not recognized as doctors and therefore unable to practice medicine), there are still NDs who can advise you on your journey if you're willing to make the drive.

Here's to your health, and God bless!

Dr Lauren

REFERENCES

References:
Chapter 1

1. Graham, Drew. "How Vegetable Oils Replaced Animal Fats in the American Diet." The Atlantic. Atlantic Media Company, 26 Apr. 2012. Web. 13 Nov. 2015. <http://www.theatlantic.com/health/archive/2012/04/how-vegetable-oils-replaced-animal-fats-in-the-american-diet/256155/>.

2. Campbell, T. Colin. The China Study: The Most Comprehensive Study of Nurtrition Ever Conducted and the Starling Implications for Diet, Weight Loss and Long-term Health. Dallas, TX.: Banbella, 2006. Print.

3. Landers, Timothy, Bevin Cohen, Thomas Wittum, and Elaine Larson. "A Review of Antibiotic Use in Food Animals: Perspective, Policy, and Po-

tential." Public Health Reports. Association of Schools of Public Health, 2012. Web. 13 Nov. 2015. <http://www.ncbi.nlm.nih.gov/pmc/articles/PM-C3234384/>.

4. "Nutrition-Related Issues." FAO. Agriculture and Consumer Protection. Web. 13 Nov. 2015. <http://www.fao.org/wairdocs/ae584e/ ae584e05.htm>.

5. Walton, Alice G. "How Much Sugar Are Americans Eating?" Forbes. Forbes Magazine, 30 Aug. 2012. Web. 13 Nov. 2015. <http://www.-forbes.com/sites/alicegwalton/2012/08/30/how-much-sugar-are-americans-eating-infographic/>.

Chapter 2

1. Washington State University. "Commercial organic farms have better fruit and soil, lower environmental impact, study finds." ScienceDaily. ScienceDaily, 2 September 2010. <www.sciencedaily.-com/releases/2010/09/100901171553.htm>.

Chapter 3

1. Obregon-Tito et al. (2015). Subsistence strategies in traditional societies distinguish gut microbiomdes. *Nat Commun* 6, 6505. Doi: 10. 1038/ ncomms7505.

2. Schnorr et al. (2014). Gut microbiome of the

Hadza hunter-gatherers. *Nat Commun*, 5, 3654. doi: 10. 1038/ncomms4654.

3. De Fillippo et al. (2010). Impact of diets in shaping gut microbiota revealed by a comparative study in children form Europe and rural Africa. *Proc Natl Acad Sci U S A*, 107(33), 14691-14696.

Chapter 4

1. Lappe, Joan M, Diane Travers-Gustafson, K Michael Davies, Robert R Recker, and Robert P Heaney. "Vitamin D and Calcium Supplementation Reduces Cancer Risk: Results of a Randomized Trial." The American Journal of Clinical Nutrition 85.6 (2007): 1586-591. Print.

2. Mead, M. "Benefits of Sunlight: A Bright Spot for Human Health." Environmental Health Perspectives. National Institute of Environmental Health Sciences, 1 Apr. 2008. Web. 13 Nov. 2015. <http://www.ncbi.nlm.nih.gov/pmc/articles/PMC2290997/>.

3. "Vitamin D Deficiency Linked More Closely to Diabetes than Obesity." Vitamin D Deficiency Linked More Closely to Diabetes than Obesity. Endocrine Society, 23 Feb. 2015. Web. 13 Nov. 2015. <https://www.endocrine.org/news-room/current-press-releases/vitamin-d-deficiency-linked-more-closely-to-diabetes-than-obesity>.

4. Munger, K. L., S. M. Zhang, E. O'reilly, M. A. Hernan, M. J. Olek, W. C. Willett, and A. Ascherio. "Vitamin D Intake and Incidence of Multiple Sclerosis." Neurology 62.1 (2004): 60-65. Penn State. American Academy of Neurology. Web. 13 Nov. 2015.

5. Pearson, Catherine. "Can Vitamin D Help With Cramps?" The Huffington Post. TheHuffingtonPost.com, 27 Feb. 2012. Web. 13 Nov. 2015. <http://www.huffingtonpost.com/2012/02/27/vitamin-d-pms-menstrual-cramps-italy_n_1305127.html>.

6. Grogan, Martha. "Calcium Supplements: A Risk Factor for Heart Attack?" *Mayo Clinic*. Mayo Foundation for Medicl Education and Research, 19 Apr. 2013. Web. 15 Nov. 2015. <http://www.mayoclinic.org/diseases-conditions/heart-attack/expert-answers/calcium-supplements/faq-20058352>

7. "Calcium beyond the Bones - Harvard Health." *Harvard Health*. Harvard Health Publications, 1 Mar. 2010. Web. 15 Nov. 2015. <http://www.health.harvard.edu/womens-health/calcium-beyond-the-bones>

8. Paddock, Catharine. "Sun Exposure Benefits May Outweigh Risks Say Scientists." Medical News Today. MediLexicon International, 8 May 2013. Web. 13 Nov. 2015. <http://www.medicalnewsto-

day.com/articles/260247.php>.

9. Mead, M. "Benefits of Sunlight: A Bright Spot for Human Health." Environmental Health Perspectives. National Institute of Environmental Health Sciences, 1 Apr. 2008. Web. 13 Nov. 2015. <http://www.ncbi.nlm.nih.gov/pmc/articles/PMC2290997/>.

Chapter 5

1. "Insufficient Sleep Is a Public Health Problem." Centers for Disease Control and Prevention. U.S. Department of Health and Human Services, 3 Sept. 2015. Web. 13 Nov. 2015. <http://www.cdc.gov/features/dssleep/>.

2. Meco, Antonio Di, Yash B. Joshi, and Domenico Praticò. "Sleep Deprivation Impairs Memory, Tau Metabolism, and Synaptic Integrity of a Mouse Model of Alzheimer's Disease with Plaques and Tangles." Neurobiology of Aging 35.8 (2014): 1813-820. Neurobiology of Aging. Elsevier. Web. 13 Nov. 2015.

3. Kawai, N., N. Sakai, M. Okuro, S. Karakawa, Y. Tsuneyoshi, N. Kawasaki, T. Takeda, M. Bannai, and S. Nishino. "The Sleep-promoting and Hypothermic Effects of Glycine Are Mediated by NMDA Receptors in the Suprachiasmatic Nucleus." National Center for Biotechnology Information. U.S. National Library of Medicine, 23 Dec. 2014. Web. 13 Nov.

2015. <http://www.ncbi.nlm.nih.gov/pubmed/
25553534>.

Chapter 7

1. Covey, Stephen R. The 7 Habits of Highly
Effective People: Powerful Lessons in Personal
Change. 25th Anniversary ed. Simon & Schuster,
2013. Print.

2. Wenner, Melinda. "Smile! It Could Make
You Happier." Scientific American Global RSS. Scientific American, 1 Aug. 2009. Web. 23 Sept. 2015.
<http://www.scientificamerican.com/article/smile-it-
could-make-you-happier>.

3. Martin, Hugo. "More than Half of Americans
Have Gone 12 Months without a Vacation." Los Angeles Times. Los Angeles Times, 13 Aug. 2015.
Web. 23 Sept. 2015. <http://www.latimes.com/busi-
ness/la-fi-12-months-without-a-vacation-20150813-
story.html>.

4. Renzulli, Kerri Anne. "How to Disconnect
from Work This Vacation." Time. Time, 18 July
2014. Web. 23 Sept. 2015. <http://time.com/money/
2982053/unplug-disconnect-work-vacation-career-
boss-email-phone/>.

5. Eaker, Elaine D., Joan Pinsky, and William P.
Castelli. "Myocardial Infarction and Coronary Death
among Women: Psychosocial Predictors from a 20-

Year Follow-up of Women in the Framingham Study." American Journal of Epidemiology 135.8 (1992): 854-64. Oxford Journals. Oxford University Press. Web. 23 Sept. 2015. <http://aje.oxfordjournals.org/content/135/8/854.short>.

6. Virtanen, Marianna, Katriina Heikkilä, Markus Jokela, Jane E. Ferrie, G. David Batty, Jussi Vahtera, and Mika Kivimäki. "Long Working Hours and Coronary Heart Disease: A Systematic Review and Meta-Analysis." American Journal of Epidemiology 176.7 (2012): 586-96. Oxford Journals. Oxford University Press. Web. 23 Sept. 2015. <http://aje.oxfordjournals.org/content/176/7/586>.

7. Virtanen M, Stansfeld SA, Fuhrer R, Ferrie JE, Kivimäki M (2012) Overtime Work as a Predictor of Major Depressive Episode: A 5-Year Follow-Up of the Whitehall II Study. PLoS ONE 7(1): e30719. doi:10.1371/journal.pone.0030719 Web. 23 Sept. 2015. <http://journals.plos.org/plosone/article?id=10.1371/journal.pone.0030719>

8. Virtanen, Marianna, Archana Singh-Manoux, Jane E. Ferrie, David Gimeno, Michael G. Marmot, Marko Elovainio, Markus Jokela, Jussi Vahtera, and Mika Kivimäki. "Long Working Hours and Cognitive Function The Whitehall II Study." American Journal of Epidemiology 169.5 (2009): 596-605. Oxford Journals. Oxford University Press. Web. 23

Sept. 2015. <10.1093/aje/kwn382>.

9. Fritz, Charlotte, and Sabine Sonnentag. "Recovery, Well-being, and Performance-related Outcomes: The Role of Workload and Vacation Experiences." Journal of Applied Psychology 91.4 (2006): 936-45. APA PsycNET. American Psychological Association. Web. 23 Sept. 2015. <http://psycnet.apa.org/journals/apl/91/4/936/>.

10. Casey, John. "Do You Know How Much Sugar You're Eating?" *MedicineNet*. MedicineNet, 16 Dec. 2003. Web. 21 Nov. 2015. <http://www.medicinenet.com/script/main/art.asp?articlekey=56589>.

Chapter 8

1. Cloud, Henry, and John Sims Townsend. Boundaries: When to Say Yes, How to Say No, to Take Control of Your Life. Zondervan, 1992. Print.

2. Boyles, Salynn. "Happiness Is Contagious." WebMD. WebMD, 4 Dec. 2008. Web. 23 Sept. 2015.

3. Gladwell, Malcolm. Outliers: The Story of Success. Little, Brown, 2008. Print.

Chapter 9

1. Maslow, Abraham H. A Theory of Human Motivation. Martino Fine, 2013. Print.

2. Ferriss, Timothy. The 4-hour Workweek: Escape 9-5, Live Anywhere, and Join the New Rich. Expanded and Updated Ed., 1st Revised ed. New York: Crown, 2009. Print.

3. Seligman, Martin E. P. Learned Optimism: How to Change Your Mind and Your Life. New York: Vintage, 2006. Print.

4. Frankl, Viktor E. Man's Search for Meaning. Boston: Beacon, 2006. Print.

5. Amen, Daniel G. Change Your Brain, Change Your Life: The Breakthrough Program for Conquering Anxiety, Depression, Obsessiveness, Anger, and Impulsiveness. New York: Times, 2000. Print.

6. Hruby, Patrick. "Washington Was Making Rep. Tim Ryan Sick ... until He Found Mindfulness." Washington Times. The Washington Times, 11 July 2012. Web. 25 Sept. 2015. <http://www.washingtontimes.com/news/2012/jul/11/ohio-democrat-uses-mindfulness-stress-reduction-te/?page=1>.

Chapter 10

1. Anand, Preetha, Ajaikumar Kunnumakara, Chitra Sundaram, Kuzhuvelil Harikumar, Sheeja Tharakan, Oiki Lai, Bokyung Sung, and Bharat Aggarwal. "Cancer Is a Preventable Disease That Requires Major Lifestyle Changes." Pharmaceutical Research. Springer US, 15 July 2008. Web. 26 Sept. 2015. <http://www.ncbi.nlm.nih.gov/pmc/articles/

PMC2515569/>.

    2. Potera, Carol. "DIET AND NUTRITION: The Artificial Food Dye Blues." Environmental Health Perspectives. National Institute of Environmental Health Sciences, 1 Oct. 2010. Web. 26 Sept. 2015. <http://www.ncbi.nlm.nih.gov/pmc/articles/PMC2957945/>.

    3. Hengel, M., and T. Shibamoto. "Carcinogenic 4(5)-methylimidazole Found in Beverages, Sauces, and Caramel Colors: Chemical Properties, Analysis, and Biological Activities." National Center for Biotechnology Information. U.S. National Library of Medicine, 15 Jan. 2013. Web. 26 Sept. 2015. <http://www.ncbi.nlm.nih.gov/pubmed/23294412>.

    4. Beaulieu, Robert, Ronald Warwar, and Bruce Buerk. "Canthaxanthin Retinopathy with Visual Loss: A Case Report and Review." Case Reports in Ophthalmological Medicine. Hindawi Publishing Corporation, 30 Oct. 2013. Web. 26 Sept. 2015. <http://www.ncbi.nlm.nih.gov/pmc/articles/PMC3833018/>.

    5. Souza, Russell, Andrew Mente, Adriana Maroleanu, Adrian Cozma, Vanessa Ha, Teruko Kishibe, Elizabeth Uleryk, Patrick Budylowski, Holger Schünemann, Joseph Beyene, and Sonia Anand. "Intake of Saturated and Trans Unsaturated Fatty Acids and Risk of All Cause Mortality, Cardiovascu-

lar Disease, and Type 2 Diabetes: Systematic Review and Meta-analysis of Observational Studies." BMJ : British Medical Journal. BMJ Publishing Group Ltd., 12 Aug. 2015. Web. 26 Sept. 2015.

6. "World Cancer Research Fund Officially Recommends Avoiding Processed Meat." CNN IReport. 22 May 2013. Web. 26 Sept. 2015. <http://ireport.cnn.com/docs/DOC-1048224>.

7. Nöthlings, U., LR Wilkens, SP Murphy, JH Hankin, BE Henderson, and LN Kolonel. "Meat and Fat Intake as Risk Factors for Pancreatic Cancer: The Multiethnic Cohort Study." National Center for Biotechnology Information. U.S. National Library of Medicine, 5 Oct. 2005. Web. 26 Sept. 2015. <http://www.ncbi.nlm.nih.gov/pubmed/16204695>.

8. "Lower Your Cancer Risk by Eating Right." Lower Your Cancer Risk by Eating Right. American Cancer Society. Web. 26 Sept. 2015. <http://www.cancer.org/myacs/newengland/lower-your-cancer-risk-by-eating-right>.

9. Ashok, Iyaswamy, and Rathinasamy Sheeladevi. "Biochemical Responses and Mitochondrial Mediated Activation of Apoptosis on Long-term Effect of Aspartame in Rat Brain." Redox Biology. Elsevier, 29 Apr. 2014. Web. 26 Sept. 2015. <http://www.ncbi.nlm.nih.gov/pmc/articles/PMC4085354/>.

10. Addicott, Merideth, Lucie Yang, Ann Peiffer,

Luke Burnett, Jonathan Burdette, Michael Chen, Satoru Hayasaka, Robert Kraft, Joseph Maldjian, and Paul Laurienti. "The Effect of Daily Caffeine Use on Cerebral Blood Flow: How Much Caffeine Can We Tolerate?" Human Brain Mapping. U.S. National Library of Medicine, 30 Oct. 2009. Web. 26 Sept. 2015. <http://www.ncbi.nlm.nih.gov/pmc/articles/ PMC2748160/>.

11. Mesnage, R., N. Defarge, J. Spiroux De Vendômois, and GE Séralini. "Potential Toxic Effects of Glyphosate and Its Commercial Formulations below Regulatory Limits." National Center for Biotechnology Information. U.S. National Library of Medicine, 12 Aug. 2015. Web. 27 Sept. 2015. <http://www.ncbi.nlm.nih.gov/pubmed/26282372>.

12. Price, Weston A. Nutrition and Physical Degeneration. 8th ed. Lemon Grove, CA: Price-Pottenger Nutrition Foundation, 2008. Print.

13. Gordon, Serena. "Link Between Diabetes, Alzheimer's Disease Strengthened." Consumer HealthDay. HealthDay, 25 Aug. 2010. Web. 26 Sept. 2015. <http://consumer.healthday.com/cognitive-and-neurological-health-information-26/alzheimer-s-news-20/link-between-diabetes-alzheimer-s-disease-strengthened-642482.html>.

14. Paddock, Catharine. "Chocolate Gorging Linked To Opium Chemical In Brain." Medical

News Today. MediLexicon International, 21 Sept. 2012. Web. 26 Sept. 2015. <http://www.medicalnewstoday.com/articles/250517.php>.

15. "Personalized Nutrition Project." *Personalized Nutrition Project*. Weizmann Institute of Science. Web. 29 Nov. 2015. <http://newsite.personalnutrition.org/WebSite/Home.aspx?study=pnp>.

16. Fowler, Sharon P.g., Ken Williams, and Helen P. Hazuda. "Diet Soda Intake Is Associated with Long-Term Increases in Waist Circumference in a Biethnic Cohort of Older Adults: The San Antonio Longitudinal Study of Aging." *Journal of the American Geriatrics Society J Am Geriatr Soc* 63.4 (2015): 708-15. *Wiley Online Library*. John Wiley & Sons, Inc. Web. 29 Nov. 2015.

17. Kobylewski, Sarah. "CSPI Says Food Dyes Pose Rainbow of Risks ~ Newsroom ~ News from CSPI ~ Center for Science in the Public Interest." CSPI Says Food Dyes Pose Rainbow of Risks ~ Newsroom ~ News from CSPI ~ Center for Science in the Public Interest. Center For Science In The Public Interest, 29 June 2010. Web. 26 Sept. 2015. <http://www.cspinet.org/new/201006291.html>.

18. Fung, Teresa, Meredith Arasaratnam, Francine Grodstein, Jeffrey Katz, Bernard Rosner, Walter Willett, and Diane Feskanich. "Soda Consumption and Risk of Hip Fractures in Post-

menopausal Women in the Nurses' Health Study." The American Journal of Clinical Nutrition. American Society for Nutrition, 6 Aug. 2014. Web. 26 Sept. 2015. <http://www.ncbi.nlm.nih.gov/pmc/articles/PMC4135502/>.

Chapter 11
1.   Tomljenovic, L., and CA Shaw. "Do Aluminum Vaccine Adjuvants Contribute to the Rising Prevalence of Autism?" National Center for Biotechnology Information. U.S. National Library of Medicine, 23 Aug. 2011. Web. 22 Oct. 2015.

Chapter 12
1.   *The Greater Good.* Dir. Kendall Nelson and Chris Pilaro. BNP Pictures, 2011. Film.
2.   Sears, Robert W. The Vaccine Book: Making the Right Decision for Your Child. New York: Little, Brown, 2007. Print.
3.   "How Common Is Autism?" *Autism Science Foundation.* Autism Science Foundation. Web. 8 Dec. 2015. <http://www.autismsciencefoundation.org/what-is-autism/how-common-is-autism>.
4.   Blumberg, Stephen J., Matthew D. Bramlett, Michael D. Kogan, Laura A. Schieve, Jessica R. Jones, and MIchael C. Lu. "Changes in Prevalence of Parent-reported Autism Spectrum Disorder in

School-aged U.S. Children: 2007 to 2011-2012." *Centers for Disease Control and Prevention.* U.S. Department of Health and Human Services, 20 Mar. 2013. Web. 8 Dec. 2015. <http://www.cdc.gov/nchs/data/nhsr/nhsr065.pdf>.

5. Valenstein, Blaming the Brain, 70-79. Also see David Healy, The Creation of Psychopharmacology (Cambridge, MA: Harvard University Press, 2002), 106, 205-206.

6. M. Bowers, "Lumbar CSF 5-hydroxyindoleacetic acid and homovanillic acid in affective syndromes," Journal of Nervous and Mental Disease 158 (1974):325-30.

7. J. Mendels, "Brain biogenic amine depletion and mood," Archives of General Psychiatry 30 (1974):447-51.

8. M. Asberg, "Serotonin depression: A biochemical subgroup within the affective disorders?" Science 191 (1976): 478-80; M. Asberg, "5-HIAA in the cerebrospinal fluid," Archives of General Psychiatry 33 (1976):1193-97.

9. J. Lacasse, "Serotonin and depression: a disconnect between the advertisements and the scientific literature," PloS Medicine 2 (2005): 1211-16.

10. C. Ross, Pseudoscience in Biological Psychiatry (New York: John Wiley & Sons, 1995),111.

11. D. Wong, "Subsensitivity of serotonin recep-

tors after long-term treatment of rats with fluoxetine," Research Communications in Chemical Pathology and Pharmacology 32 (1981):41-51.

12. J. Wamsley, "Receptor alterations associated with serotonergic agents," Journal of Clinical Psychiatry 48, suppl. (1987):19-25.

13. C. Silverman, The Epidemiology of Depression (Baltimore: Johns Hopkins Press, 1968), 139.

14. Social Security Administration, annual statistical reports on the SSI program, 1996-2008; and Social Security Bulletin, Annual Statistical Supplement, 1988-1992.

15. U.S. Government Accountability Office, "Young adults with serious mental illness" (June 2008).

16. K. Solomon, "Pitfalls and prospects in clinical research on antianxiety drugs," Journal of Clinical Psychiatry 39 (1978):823-31.

17. H. Ashton, "Protracted withdrawal syndromes from benzodiazepines," Journal of Substance Abuse Treatment 9 (1991):19-28.

18. A. Pelissolo, "Anxiety and depressive disorders in 4,425 long term benzodiazepine users in general practice," Encephale 33 (2007):32-38

19. Schuyler, The Depressive Spectrum, 47

20. G. Fava, "Can long-term treatment with antidepressant drugs worsen the course of depression?"

Journal of Clinical Psychiatry 64 (2003):123-33.

21. W. Coryell, "Characteristics and significance of untreated major depressive disorder," American Journal of Psychiatry 152 (1995):1124-29.

22. A. Zis, "Major affective disorder as a recurrent illness," Archives of General Psychiatry 36 (1979):835-39.

23. Social Security Administration, annual statistical reports on the SSDI and SSI programs, 1987-2008.

24. M. Barker, "Cognitive effects of long-term benzodiazepine use," CNS Drugs 18 (2004):37-48.

25. Government Accountability Office, Young Adults with Serious Mental Illness, June 2008.

26. "Yasmin Side Effects in Detail." Drugs.com. Drugs.com. Web. 22 Oct. 2015.

27. Weschler, Toni. Taking Charge of Your Fertility: The Definitive Guide to Natural Birth Control, Pregnancy Achievement, and Reproductive Health. 20th Anniversary Edition, First ed. William Morrow Paperbacks, 2015. Print.

Chapter 14

1. Gottschall, Elaine Gloria. Breaking the Vicious Cycle: Intestinal Health through Diet. Kirkton, Ont.: Kirkton, 1994. Print.

* * *

Chapter 15
   1. "Fasting Triggers Stem Cell Regeneration of Damaged, Old Immune System." EurekAlert! American Association for the Advancement of Science, 5 June 2014. Web. 24 Oct. 2015.

Chapter 17
   1. Colquhoun, J. "New Evidence on Fluoridation." National Center for Biotechnology Information. U.S. National Library of Medicine, 1984. Web. 27 Oct. 2015.
   2. Pavelka, S., A. Babický, M. Vobecký, and J. Lener. "Effect of High Bromide Levels in the Organism on the Biological Half-life of Iodine in the Rat." National Center for Biotechnology Information. U.S. National Library of Medicine, 2001. Web. 27 Oct. 2015.
   3. Van Leeuwen, FX, and B. Sangster. "The Toxicology of Bromide Ion." National Center for Biotechnology Information. U.S. National Library of Medicine, 1987. Web. 27 Oct. 2015.
   4. Ain, KB, Y. Mori, and S. Refetoff. "Reduced Clearance Rate of Thyroxine-binding Globulin (TBG) with Increased Sialylation: A Mechanism for Estrogen-induced Elevation of Serum TBG Concentration." National Center for Biotechnology Information. U.S. National Library of Medicine, 1 Oct. 1987.

Web. 27 Oct. 2015.

5. Gerli, S., E. Papaleo, A. Ferrari, and GC Di Renzo. "Randomized, Double Blind Placebo-controlled Trial: Effects of Myo-inositol on Ovarian Function and Metabolic Factors in Women with PCOS." National Center for Biotechnology Information. U.S. National Library of Medicine, 1 Sept. 2007. Web. 27 Oct. 2015.

6. Costantino, D., G. Minozzi, F. Minozzi, and C. Guaraldi. "Metabolic and Hormonal Effects of Myo-inositol in Women with Polycystic Ovary Syndrome: A Double-blind Trial." Eur Rev Med Pharmacol Sci 13.N. 2: 105-10. Print.

7. Raffone, E., P. Rizzo, and V. Benedetto. "Insulin Sensitiser Agents Alone and in Co-treatment with R-FSH for Ovulation Induction in PCOS Women." National Center for Biotechnology Information. U.S. National Library of Medicine, 26 Apr. 2010. Web. 27 Oct. 2015.

8. "Generational Decline in Testosterone Levels Observed." Healio. Endocrine Today, 1 Feb. 2007. Web. 27 Oct. 2015.

9. Patterson, TR, JD Stringham, and AW Meikle. "Nicotine and Cotinine Inhibit Steroidogenesis in Mouse Leydig Cells." National Center for Biotechnology Information. U.S. National Library of Medicine, 1990. Web. 27 Oct. 2015.

10. Lucero, J., BL Harlow, RL Barbieri, P. Sluss, and DW Cramer. "Early Follicular Phase Hormone Levels in Relation to Patterns of Alcohol, Tobacco, and Coffee Use." National Center for Biotechnology Information. U.S. National Library of Medicine, 1 Oct. 2001. Web. 27 Oct. 2015.

11. Ferrini, Rebecca L., and Elizabeth Barrett-Connor. "Caffeine Intake and EndogenousSex Sterois Levels in Postmenopausal Women." American Journal of Epidemiology (1996): 642-44. Print.

GLOSSARY

5-alpha reductase: The enzyme that converts testosterone into dihydrotestosterone (DHT), thus partly responsible for conditions such as BPH (Benign Prostatic Hypertrophy), male pattern hair loss, hirsuitism, and acne.

Acupuncture: An ancient medical practice adhering to Traditional Chinese Medicine principles, involving needles strategically placed in the body along meridians corresponding to the function of internal organs.

Adrenaline: Also known as epinephrine, adrenaline is the "fight or flight" hormone. It causes your heart to race, your bronchioles to dilate, and provides your muscles with immediate blood flow (oxygen and

426

glucose for energy) to get away quickly or fight.

Adrenals: two pyramid- shaped glands that sit on top of your kidneys and produce hormones to help your body cope with stress.

Aldosterone: A hormone produced by the adrenals that reabsorbs sodium and exchanges it for potassium in the kidneys. Water follows sodium, so as you reabsorb sodium, you reabsorb water also, which means aldosterone helps to regulate blood volume.

Amino acids: The twenty biochemical building blocks for proteins.

Androgens: Hormones in the testosterone family, including DHEA, testosterone, dihydrotestosterone (DHT), and androstenedione.

Anovulatory cycles: menstrual cycles during which a woman does not ovulate.

Antigens: substances that have the potential to provoke your specific immune system to make antibodies against them. Soluble antigens come from your diet and your environment; insoluble antigens come from microbes and pathogens; and self antigens come from your own cells.

Antioxidants: nutrients that neutralize or quench free radicals (unpaired electrons) which can cause oxidative stress.

Aromitase: an enzyme that resides in fat cells and converts testosterone into estrogen.

ATP: Adenosine Triphosphate, the main energy currency in the human body, produced inside mitochondrial cells.

B cells: immune cells that produce antibodies against antigens, and are directed by T cells.

Benzodiazepines: currently the most popular type of anti-anxiety medication, which work by stimulating the GABA receptors. I often abbreviate them "benzos".

Bioavailable: molecules that are not bound to binding globulins, and thus are able to be used by the body for their purpose (to be absorbed, to stimulate receptors, etc).

Botanical: made from herbs.

Candida: an opportunistic fungal organism which, when overgrown, can cause symptoms such as gas, bloating, itchy ears, brain fog, rashes, thrush, constipation and diarrhea.

Canola oil: an oil marketed as a health food, which is made from rapeseed, is often genetically modified, and is very high in inflammatory omega 6 fatty acids.

Carbohydrates: one of the three human macronutrients (the other two are protein and fat); of the three, it is most easily converted into glucose and energy.

Carcinogen: A substance known to cause cancer.

Castor oil packs: Part of a detox protocol which brings more blood flow to the liver, encouraging faster waste elimination than would happen physiologically.

Celiac Disease: an autoimmune disease in which gluten proteins trigger the production of antibodies against the small intestine villi.

Chelated mineral forms: Negatively charged ions

which bind to minerals your body needs loosely enough to release them easily for absorption.

Cholesterol: cholesterol is a carrier for fat. Fat gets stored as triglycerides, and triglycerides get packaged into either HDL (High Density Lipoproteins) or LDL (Low Density Lipoproteins), depending on whether they're headed to your liver to get broken down and used as energy, or whether they're headed from your liver to the rest of you to get stored as fat (respectively).

Codependency: Taking responsibility for something that is rightfully another person's problem, or allowing someone else to take responsibility for something that is rightfully yours.

Colon hydrotherapy: irrigation of the colon with water, high enough to trigger dumping of bile into the colon for the purpose of detoxification. Usually the process takes about an hour from a licensed colon hydrotherapist.

Cottonseed oil: an oil marketed as a health food, which is made from cottonseed, is often genetically modified, and is very high in inflammatory omega 6 fatty acids.

Cortisol: a hormone that encourages the breakdown of glycogen (stored glucose) and gluconeogenesis (production of new glucose from fat in the liver). It redirects blood flow to repair tissues and digest food, it's anti-inflammatory, and an immune suppressant.

Cruciferous vegetables: the veggies that "flower outward"— like broccoli, cauliflower, bok choy, and brussels sprouts. These are excellent support for liver detoxification.

Cytochrome systems: Phase 1 Detoxification queues to break down specific types of foreign chemicals, hormones, and toxins.

DHEA (Dehydroepiandrosterone): DHEA is one of three major cholesterol-based hormones produced by your adrenal glands, along with aldosterone and cortisol. DHEA is a precursor hormone for estrogen and testosterone in both men and women.

Dihydrotestosterone (DHT): a metabolite of testosterone in the androgen family, partly responsible for conditions such as BPH (Benign Prostatic Hypertrophy), male pattern hair loss, hirsuitism, and acne.

Dirty Dozen: The twelve fruits and veggies ranked yearly by the Environmental Working Group as the most contaminated with pesticides. (http://www.ewg.org/foodnews/ summary/)

Dopamine: The neurotransmitter most often associated with the nucleus accumbens, the "pleasure center" of the brain; deficiencies are characteristic of Parkinson's Disease, and excesses are implicated in anxiety and OCD.

Dry skin brushing: brushing your skin from the outer limbs towards the body's core to follow the line of lymphatic drainage, helping to flush toxins into organs of elimination.

Dysbiosis: a general term for imbalance of gut flora.

Electrolyte: The word electrolyte generally refers to the largest concentration of charged particles within the human body. The biggest two are sodium and chloride. Others include magnesium and potassium.

Endocrine: another word for hormones.

Endorphins: the neurotransmitters released with

certain stimuli including exercise. They are chemically to morphine, and can decrease sensitivity to pain and even induce euphoria.

Enriched: A term on food labels meaning that vitamins and minerals that were lost during processing and were added back.

Enzymes: compounds that act like pairs of scissors in your digestive tract, to cut bigger molecules into smaller pieces. Different types of food require different enzymes.

Estrogen: The primary female hormone, which primarily acts to stimulate proliferation (particularly of the uterine lining during the first half of a woman's menstrual cycle).

Estrogen dominance: an excess of estrogen relative to progesterone; it can mean either that estrogen levels are high, or that progesterone levels are low. Symptoms include irritability , weepiness, anxiety , depression, mood swings, breast tenderness, severe menstrual cramping, heavy, prolonged bleeding (menorrhagia), spotting between cycles, thick clotting in menstrual blood, acne, hot flashes and night sweats, water retention, fibrocystic breasts, fibroids, migraines, and endometriosis.

Essential fatty acids: the most beneficial type of fat, essential because you have to get them from your diet. They're anti-inflammatory, they support the mucus lining in your stomach, lower blood pressure and cholesterol, improve insulin sensitivity , decrease allergic responses, keep cell walls healthy, and are necessary for brain development.

Fasting: skipping meals for a period of time in order to allow your body to reallocate the energy it might have used on digestion to instead help your body to heal.

Fat: One of the three macronutrients (the other two are carbohydrates and protein); a nonpolar molecule with a carbon backbone bonded to hydrogens. It is an efficient storage method for energy.

Fermented/Fermentation: fermentation happens in the absence of oxygen, and it's the conversion of carbohydrates (sugar) to alcohol or lactic acid, and carbon dioxide (CO_2).

Ferritin: the storage form of iron, primarily in the liver, but also found in hair follicles.

Genetically Modified Organisms (GMOs): Genetic modification in general involves taking a gene from one organism, clipping it out of that organism's genome (splicing it) and then inserting it into the genome of a different organism. GMO crops usually have the pesticide glyphosate inserted directly into the plant's genome.

Ghrelin: the hormone your body releases to tell you you're hungry.

Gluconeogenesis: production of new glucose from fat in the liver.

Glucose: also called blood sugar; the precursor for the biochemical processes by which your body produces ATP, its main energy currency.

Gluten: Gluten is a protein found in the germ (see above) of wheat, rye, barley, and several other grains. It's the glue, or the core binding element, of certain grains (including wheat of course, plus barley, bulgar, couscous, durum, rye, semolina, spelt, and triticale).

Glycemic index: The glycemic index is a measure of

how quickly a particular food turns to sugar in the body. Glucose is assigned a glycemic index of 100, and everything else is assigned a number relative to that.

Glycogen: a storage form of glucose.

Goiter: an enlarged thyroid, usually associated with hypothyroidism, though it can occasionally be associated with thyroiditis or Grave's Disease.

Goitrogens: foods considered to be thyroid suppressants, because they compete with thyroid hormone for iodine. These foods include millet, peanuts, radishes, turnips, and raw cruciferous veggies (such as cauliflower, brussels sprouts, and broccoli).

Grass-fed: animal products from animals who have consumed their natural diet of grass, rather than the agriculture industry meal of grain.

Halides: elements on the periodic table in the same column as iodine, including bromine, fluorine, and chlorine. Their shared grouping means they have chemically similar behavior, and they can act as competitive inhibitors with iodine.

Heterozygous: We have two copies of every gene, one from each parent. Someone who is heterozygous for a particular gene mutation has only one copy of the mutation, as opposed to homozygous, a person who has two copies.

Hirsuitism: abnormal masculine hair growth patterns in a female.

Homeopathy/Homeopathic: Based on the principle of "like cures like," homeopathy is energetic medicine which gives the body a small "push" in the direction it's already headed. Because the body is a living system and seeks to create balance, or homeostasis, the body will self-correct in the opposite direction: back towards health.

Homozygous: We have two copies of every gene, one from each parent. Someone who is heterozygous for a particular gene mutation has only one copy of the mutation, as opposed to homozygous, a person who has two copies.

HPA (Hypothalamus-Pituitary-Adrenal) axis: The three endocrine glands that work together for the purposes of stress management. The first two are in the brain, while the adrenal glands are on top of the kidneys.

Hormones: chemical compounds that set of signaling cascades in the body.

Hormone receptors: If the hormones are the "key," receptors are the "lock" they fit into in order to begin their appropriate signal cascade.

Hydrogenation: bombarding the unsaturated (liquid) fat with hydrogen ions in order to make it saturated. The process produces trans fats, or partially hydrogenated fats.

Hydrotherapy: the therapeutic use of water. More particularly, water's specific heat makes it a great vehicle to apply alternating temperatures to the body in a variety of ways.

Hypertension: high blood pressure.

Hypoglycemia: low blood sugar.

Hypothyroidism: low thyroid function.

Hypoxia: lack of oxygen.

* * *

IgG food allergies: Allergies that have a 72 hour window in the body. This means you can eat something to which you are sensitive, and not react to it for a few days.

Inflammation: Activation of the non-specific immune system to release chemical warfare against potential invaders, leading to collateral damage of the body's tissues.

Insulin: the hormone "key" that allows glucose to exit the bloodstream and enter the cells. It is produced in the pancreas.

Intestinal permeability: aka leaky gut syndrome. Gut inflammation can disrupt the tight junctions in the small intestine, allowing food particles to come in contact with the bloodstream prematurely. This triggers the formation of IgG antibodies against foods, generally those most commonly eaten.

Irritable Bowel Disease: aka IBD, these are autoimmune conditions of the gut including Crohn's Disease and Ulcerative Colitis. Both are characterized by GI inflammation, and blood and/or mucus in the stool.

Irritable Bowel Syndrome: This is not so much a diagnosis as a description of symptoms, including gas, bloating, alternating constipation and diarrhea. There are a number of possible causes.

Juicing: removing the fiber of fruits and veggies with a juicer, leaving only the juice. This delivers

Leaky Gut Syndrome: aka intestinal permeability. Gut inflammation can disrupt the tight junctions in the small intestine, allowing food particles to come in contact with the bloodstream prematurely. This triggers the formation of IgG antibodies against foods, generally those most commonly eaten.

Leptin: the "satiety" hormone, which tells your body you're full and to stop eating.

Lymphatic circulation: recycled blood plasma. Your lymph is necessary for the immune system to remove waste, toxins, pathogens, and cancer cells.

Melatonin: the "sleep hormone", opposed to cortisol. It is also a powerful antioxidant.

* * *

Metabolic syndrome: Increased abdominal weight, cholesterol, and blood sugar, often associated with insulin resistance.

Microbiome: the collective term for all the bacteria that populate your gut—all 100 trillion of them.

Monounsaturated Fats: fats that have only a single double bond in the hydrogen chain.

Mycotoxins: mold toxins.

Neuroplasticity: the reorganization of the brain's structure when both learning something new and consolidating that memory.

Neurotoxin: a chemical that is toxic to the neurological system.

Neurotransmitters: chemical messengers in the brain.

Organic: foods grown in organic fertilizers, created from "natural" substances. These include things like compost, animal manure or guano, blood meal (from powdered blood), fish meal (from ground up fish), bone meal, etc. Usually grown with much fewer pesticides as well.

Parabens: preservatives that mimic estrogens, appearing in personal care products and associated with endocrine cancers.

Partially Hydrogenated Oils: aka trans fats. These fats have hydrogens on opposite sides of the carbon chain instead of on the same side. This means fats won't lay flat against each other, the way natural saturated fats do. If trans fats get into your cell membranes, it means signals don't get in and out of the cells very efficiently. It also means nutrients and oxygen can't get in easily, nor can metabolic waste get out.

Peristalsis: electrical signals throughout the digestive tract, pushing food downward in rhythmic waves.

Polycystic Ovarian Syndrome (PCOS): multiple ovarian cysts, which can lead to anovulation, insulin resistance, and/or androgen overproduction.

Polyunsaturated vegetable oils: fats with more than one double bond in the carbon backbone, generally high in inflammatory omega 6 fatty acids. These include canola oil, corn oil, cottonseed oil, safflower and sunflower oil.

Progesterone: Progesterone helps to prepare the uterine lining for implantation, and so it begins to rise just after ovulation. Progesterone and estrogen decline together throughout the second half of a woman's menstrual cycle, and if the two are in balance, the symptoms associated with estrogen dominance should not occur.

Protein: One of the three macronutrients (the other two are carbohydrates and fats). All of your cells are made up of proteins. Protein, in turn, is made up of amino acids (twenty of them, to be exact). Your DNA codes for each one of those individual amino acids and, like beads on a chain, your cells assemble the amino acids in sequence such that proteins can be formed.

Phthalates: Phthalates are chemicals found in flexible plastic, and are not only estrogenic, they have been found to increase programmed cell death (particularly in testicular cells). Overall, phthalates are linked to breast cancer, birth defects, low sperm count, obesity, diabetes, and thyroid problems.

Phytoestrogens: Phytoestrogens are 100 to 1000 times weaker than the estrogen your body produces naturally. Both types of molecules bind to estrogen receptors, however.

Salivary cortisol: A test to determine the rhythm of cortisol throughout the day, involving spitting into a test tube four times throughout the day.

Saturated fat: a fat whose backbone is fully saturated with hydrogens. Saturated fat makes up 50% of your cell membranes (and healthy cell membranes means good stuff can in, and bad stuff can get out). They are also the preferred food for your heart, they're antimicrobial, they support immune function, they are necessary for your blood to clot and for your lungs to work properly, they are easily absorbed for quick energy, and they are necessary for infant brain development.

Selective Serotonin Reuptake Inhibitors (SSRIs): The most popular class of drugs for depression. They prevent serotonin from getting broken down, so that they stick around in the synaptic cleft to stimulate receptors longer. These include sertraline (Zoloft), citalopram (Celexa), etc.

* * *

Small Intestine Bacterial Overgrowth (SIBO): A condition in which gut flora that is supposed to stay in the colon has crawled back into the small intestine, leading to gas, bloating, abdominal pain and cramps, both constipation and diarrhea, and stools ribboned with mucus.

Solvents: soluble chemicals that tend to get stored in human fat cells (adipose tissue) after exposure.

Specific Carbohydrate Diet: A diet plan originally designed for people with Irritable Bowel Disease by Elaine Gottschall, popularized by the book, "Breaking the Vicious Cycle." The diet avoids certain specific carbohydrates known to exacerbate the process, and also works well for SIBO.

Stem cells: undifferentiated cells which have the potential to become a wide variety of possible cells.

T cells: The director cells of the specific immune system; T cells direct the B cells to produce immunoglobulins against antigens.

T3: The active thyroid hormone, called 3 because it has only three iodine molecules attached to it. It gets converted from T4 to T3 in the peripheral tissues and in the liver.

T4: The thyroid hormone your thyroid produces in response to TSH (Thyroid Stimulating Hormone) produced from your brain. It's about 80% inactive, 20% active. It travels to your tissues and gets converted into the more active T3.

TBG: Thyroid Binding Globulin. This is the binding globulin that binds thyroid hormones, thus preventing them from stimulating thyroid receptors. Too much of this, and you can be functionally hypothyroid even if all labs look normal. It's a big reason why it's a good idea to measure the free versions of T3 and T4, rather than the total numbers.

Testosterone: The primary male sex hormone, derived from cholesterol. Testosterone contributes to a healthy libido, a sense of well-being and vitality, and healthy bones and muscles.

Thimerosol: the vaccine adjuvant (additive) containing mercury, which has been removed from most, but not all, vaccines.

Trans fats: aka Partially Hydrogenated Fats. These

fats have hydrogens on opposite sides of the carbon chain instead of on the same side. This means fats won't lay flat against each other, the way natural saturated fats do. If trans fats get into your cell membranes, it means signals don't get in and out of the cells very efficiently. It also means nutrients and oxygen can't get in easily, nor can metabolic waste get out.

Triglycerides: fats are carbon backbones with hydrogens attached to them. When your body wants to store them, they have to attach them to a glycerol backbone with three glycerol molecules, each of which can attach to one fat molecule. These triglycerides are what get stored inside your cholesterol, and delivered to either your tissues to get stored for later use, or to your liver to get broken down and turned into glucose for energy.

TSH: Thyroid Stimulating Hormone. This is the hormone produced by your pituitary gland in your brain, which tells your thyroid to produce T4. When your thyroid isn't paying enough attention and producing as well as it should (i.e. hypothyroidism), TSH tends to go up. When your thyroid is overproducing (i.e. hyperthyroidism), or when you are overmedicated, TSH tends to go down.

* * *

Volatile organic compound (VOC): chemicals that are carbon based (hence, organic) and evaporate at room temperature, which means you can breathe them in.

ABOUT THE AUTHOR

Dr. Lauren Deville is board-certified to practice medicine in the State of Arizona. She received her NMD from Southwest College of Naturopathic Medicine in Tempe, AZ, and she holds a BS in Biochemistry and Molecular Biophysics from the University of Arizona, with minors in Spanish and Creative Writing. She stumbled upon SCNM almost by accident, but the moment she walked in the doors of her future medical school, she knew that this was what she had been searching for all along. She considers herself incredibly blessed to have found a career that is also a calling.

***

Printed in Great Britain
by Amazon

44096680R00270